Understanding Diverticular Health: A Comprehensive Guide

Carolinex P. Thomas

All rights reserved.
Copyright © 2023 Carolinex P. Thomas

COPYRIGHT © 2023 Carolinex P. Thomas

All rights reserved.

No part of this book must be reproduced, stored in a retrieval system, or shared by any means, electronic, mechanical, photocopying, recording, or otherwise, without written permission from the publisher.

Every precaution has been taken in the preparation of this book; still the publisher and author assume no responsibility for errors or omissions. Nor do they assume any liability for damages resulting from the use of the information contained herein.

Legal Notice:

This book is copyright protected and is only meant for your individual use. You are not allowed to amend, distribute, sell, use, quote or paraphrase any of its part without the written consent of the author or publisher.

Introduction

In this comprehensive guide, we will delve into the intricacies of these gastrointestinal conditions and explore the various aspects of managing them through a specialized diet. Whether you've been diagnosed with diverticulitis or diverticulosis or are seeking preventive measures, this guide will serve as your go-to resource for understanding, preventing, and managing these conditions effectively.

To begin our journey, we will take a closer look at how the gut works, providing you with a foundational understanding of the digestive system. This knowledge will help you grasp the intricate processes involved and how they relate to diverticulitis and diverticulosis.

Next, we will dive into the specifics of diverticulitis, shedding light on what it is and how it differs from diverticulosis. Understanding the nature of diverticulitis will allow you to comprehend the challenges it presents and the measures required to alleviate its symptoms.

In our exploration of diverticulitis, we will also investigate the underlying causes of this condition. Identifying these causes is crucial for developing effective strategies to manage and prevent diverticulitis. By gaining insight into the factors that contribute to its development, you can make informed decisions about your lifestyle and dietary choices.

The guide will also discuss the symptoms associated with diverticulitis, allowing you to recognize and differentiate them from other gastrointestinal conditions. Recognizing the symptoms is essential for timely diagnosis and appropriate management.

Speaking of diagnosis, we will delve into the various methods used to diagnose diverticulitis. Equipped with this knowledge, you will understand the procedures and tests involved, enabling you to actively participate in your healthcare journey.

Prevention plays a vital role in managing diverticulitis and preventing flare-ups. We will explore practical strategies and lifestyle modifications that can help prevent the occurrence of diverticulitis attacks. By implementing these measures, you can reduce the frequency and severity of symptoms.

In cases where surgery becomes necessary, we will discuss the surgeries used to remove diverticulitis. Understanding the surgical options and advancements in this field will provide you with valuable insights into potential treatment paths.

As we progress through the guide, we will touch upon recent advancements in science related to diverticulitis. Keeping abreast of the latest research and breakthroughs allows you to stay informed about emerging treatments and management strategies.

We value your input and invite you to help shape our book. Your feedback and experiences are invaluable, and we encourage you to actively participate in refining the content to ensure it meets your needs and expectations.

Finally, we will provide you with a collection of recipes tailored to different stages of diverticulitis and diverticulosis management. From meals to enjoy during flare-ups to a diverticulitis prevention diet, our diverse range of recipes will support your dietary needs throughout the day, from breakfast to lunch and dinner.

Join us on this journey to better understand and manage diverticulitis and diverticulosis. Together, we will explore the intricacies of these conditions and discover the power of a specialized diet in promoting digestive health and overall well-being. Let's embark on this transformative path towards a healthier gut and a better quality of life.

Contents

How the Gut Works 1
What is Diverticulitis? 4
What Causes Diverticulitis? 7
Symptoms Associated with Diverticulitis 12
Diagnosing Diverticulitis 14
How to Prevent Diverticulitis and its Attacks 17
Surgeries to Remove Diverticulitis 23
Recent Advancements in Science 25
Help Shape Our Books 47
Recipes 48
    During A Flare-Up or Acute Pain 48
    Diverticulitis Prevention Diet 49
Breakfast 51
Lunch 68
Dinner 100

How the Gut Works

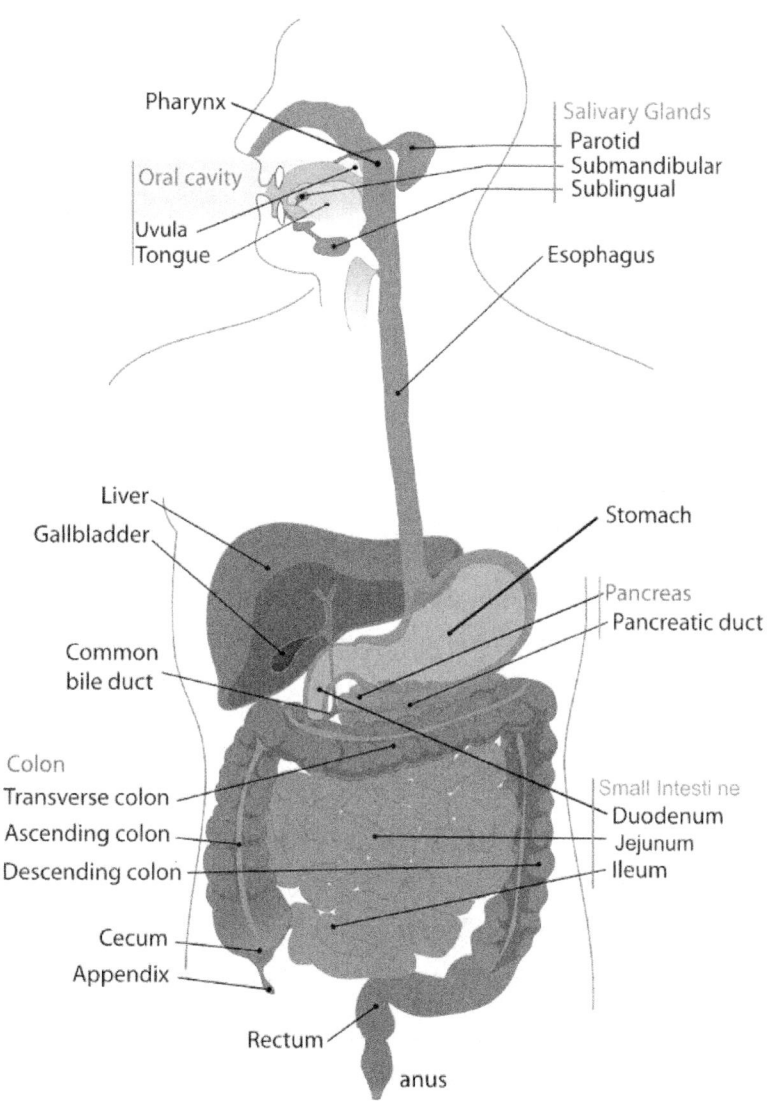

First things first, it is beneficial to gain a wider understanding of how the gut works in its entirety. If you are already well-versed in how the gut operates and strictly want to know about a specific disorder, feel free to skip this part.

The digestive system starts to work from the moment food reaches your mouth and ends when it leaves your body. Food travels through a long tube with many twists and turns, being pushed through a series of processes that allow the body to absorb nutrients and remove waste. This tube is known by various names such as the alimentary canal, the gastrointestinal tract (GI tract/GIT), the digestive tract or the gut. The gut starts at the oral cavity (the mouth) and continues into the pharynx, esophagus, stomach, small intestine and finally the large intestine (which comprises of the cecum, colon, rectum and anal canal).

The process of digestion begins as soon as food enters the mouth. The food is broken into smaller particles and mixed with salivary enzymes when we chew. This concoction is then passed into the stomach. The stomach introduces new enzymes that are coupled with its highly acidic environment to break food into smaller subunits and is also used as a tank for storage, allowing the rest of the gut to finish its processes if the body has consumed a lot of food. The proteins, carbohydrates, fats and other such components are broken down into their small sub-units such as peptides/amino acids, sugars, and lipids respectively. These smaller sub-units are used to produce energy for our daily activities and contribute to our bodily maintenance.

These nutrients are then passed into the small intestine, which is where most of our nutrients are absorbed. Further enzymes from the pancreas and bile from the liver are then squeezed through ducts into the small intestine. The small intestine is made up of specialized cells that are adept at absorbing nutrients as food passes through. These nutrients are then transferred into the bloodstream, where they are sent throughout the body for use by various organs. The waste product is then passed into the large intestine, which absorbs any remaining nutrients and water and then flushes the remaining waste out of the system.

Therefore, the intestines play a central role in the process of digesting and absorbing nutrients and distributing them to the rest of the body. It is important that the walls of the intestines remain intact so that the exchange of nutrients between the intestines and the body can be controlled precisely. The intestine is also home to billions of beneficial micro-organisms that help to digest the food we eat. You may have heard of these micro-organisms by their various aliases: microflora, microbiota, microbiome or simply, good gut bacteria. Some bacteria are heavily relied upon to produce enzymes to break down carbohydrates that the body cannot.

People suffering with digestive disorders can disrupt their digestive system and upset the balance of the microflora ecosystem. These people are more susceptible to other diseases such as Small Intestinal Bacterial Overgrowth.

What is Diverticulitis?

Diverticular disease is split into two major stages: Diverticulosis and Diverticulitis. Diverticulosis is a condition characterized by tiny pouches along the large intestine known as diverticula, or diverticulum if only one is present. These tiny pouches are created by the strain of passing hard stools through the large intestine. Therefore, older people are more susceptible to this disease, as the intestines weaken with age[5].

A recent scientific review of current diverticular disease classifications has broken this into three in-depth stages; Uncomplicated Disease, Chronic Complicated Disease & Acute Complicated Disease. Acute Complicated Disease has 4 sub-classifications, these can be seen below[3]. For the purposes of simplification, this book will discuss diverticular disease in the two major stages, diverticulosis and diverticulitis, as they are common terms that doctors use.

Uncomplicated Disease

Pain in lower left quadrant, fever, changes in relief pattern.

Chronic Complicated Disease

Impaired passage of stool, recurrent rectal blood loss, incapacitating complaints, high-risk patients, fistula (abnormal connection between two body parts).

Acute Complicated Disease

1. Fever & painful mass
2. Painful obstruction of the intestine
3. Massive rectal blood loss
4. Generalized peritonitis (inflammation of the thin tissue in the inner wall of the abdomen)

    Diverticulitis occurs after these bulges become severely irritated and inflamed, turning into pouches. Diverticulitis is the main stage of this disease; luckily, most people experiencing Diverticulosis will not experience Diverticulitis. During Diverticulitis, several nasty things can happen to the diverticula. Bacteria can become trapped inside the pouches; abscesses can form in the intestines; and stool may also get lodged inside a pouch. None of these problems sound typically minor but fortunately, most people will find that these symptoms do not happen to them and the typical pain caused by Diverticulitis could be mistakenly considered to be indigestion. Therefore, it's vital to make sure someone that suffers with Diverticulitis or even Diverticulosis does everything they can to prevent inflammation and irritation to diverticula. This can mean anything from including or removing foods from their everyday diet, right up to a complete lifestyle change. In fact, scientists were able to reproduce diverticulosis in an experiment by feeding rabbits a specific diet[4]. Not only can positive lifestyle changes grant better health overall, it can reduce the chance of developing Diverticulitis.

If you are experiencing Diverticulosis you are not alone. In fact, it is estimated that 5% of people have a diverticulum by the time they reach 40 years old and 50% of people will have them by the time they are 80 years old[5]. In England, during 2010 there were roughly 80,000 hospital admissions alone[6]. Although both men and women are equally likely to suffer from this disease, men under 50 years old are more likely to experience it than women. Interestingly, diverticular disease is often described as a 'western disease' because of the exceptionally high amount of cases found in Europe and North America and the low amount of cases in African and Asian countries. This is why diet and genes are considered to be the biggest factor in acquiring this disease, often linking it to the lower fiber intake in western countries[6]. However, this view has yet to be irrefutably proven.

What Causes Diverticulitis?

Diverticulitis is an extremely difficult disease to discuss. It's so common yet the exact causation isn't entirely understood. The medical community has largely attributed it to, simply, genetics and age[5]. Unfortunately, the main triggers are two things that cannot be altered. However, there have been some particularly interesting insights into this field. Below is a list of possible causes for the triggering of this disease.

Genetics

As previously mentioned, western people are more susceptible to developing this disease. Interestingly, people that live in western countries normally develop Diverticulosis in the last third of the colon, while the relatively few people in Asian countries (such as Japan, Taiwan and Singapore) that also suffer, seem to develop Diverticulosis in the first section of the colon. It has also been noted that the Japanese population living in Hawaii are at a higher risk of Diverticulosis than those living in Japan, but they still develop it in the 'Japanese' location; which is the first part of the colon[7].

Age

Age is commonly linked to Diverticulitis because of the continual weakening of the intestines throughout their use[5].

The figures correlate directly with age; the older you are, the more chance you have of suffering from Diverticulitis. Although the link is very simple to make, it is possible that the actual cause isn't as straightforward as linking one number to another and proclaiming diverticular disease is inevitable.

Straining & Fiber

Since diverticula can be caused by increased pressure when items pass through the intestine, it is entirely possible that people experiencing frequent constipation are prone to Diverticulosis. Constipation is defined by the National Digestive Diseases Information Clearinghouse (NDDIC) of the U.S. to be: "a condition in which an adult has fewer than three bowel movements a week or has bowel movements with stools that are hard, dry, and small, making them painful or difficult to pass"[8].

We normally associate constipation with the inability to have bowel movements. Using the definition above, it is entirely possible to have constipation with frequent bowel movements, but with harder than normal stools. Diets high in fiber help to soften stools. Scientists were able to replicate Diverticulosis by feeding rabbits a refined diet of "white bread, butter, sugar, milk and vitamin supplements" providing further evidence that low fiber is a major cause[4].

Inflammation

Inflammation is "osmotically-mediated edema of catabolic origin", or in other words, fluid (red and white blood cells etc.) based swelling caused by the breakdown of cells[9]. The most obvious type of inflammation is external and occurs when irritation or injury happens to the skin. Inflammation is the body's immune system activating its self-defense which consists of a complex chain of events[10]. The body releases various substances and hormones which cause blood vessels to dilate, allowing more blood to reach the area. More blood flow means the skin becomes red and warm, simultaneously allowing more immune system cells to travel with the blood to the skin. Some of the substances the body produces possess a secondary function that makes it easier for the immune system cells to pass out of the blood vessels, allowing a greater number to reach the skin. These immune system cells cause more fluid to enter the tissue, causing it to swell. Finally, the hormones released earlier irritate the nearby nerves, causing pain signals which makes the patient protect the area from further harm. External inflammation and Internal inflammation go through the same process, but since you can't see the swelling or redness, it is often difficult to know that it's happening at all.

    Inflammation to the intestinal wall can cause Diverticulosis and aggravate diverticula, even rupturing it. Although it is widely accepted that moderate inflammation is dangerous to those suffering with Diverticulosis, chronic low-grade inflammation can also cause Diverticulosis. Approximately 75% of a 930-patient study that undertook surgery for diverticular disease showed signs of chronic inflammation around diverticula[11].

What causes inflammation of the intestinal wall? Other gut disorders such as IBS, Small Intestinal Bacterial Overgrowth and Leaky Gut Syndrome can contribute to an irritated gut lining. Non-steroidal anti-inflammatory drugs (NSAIDs), such as ibuprofen are also known to cause complications. High levels of stress have been well documented to cause a variety of negative affects to the intestines, one of which is inflammation[12]. An overconsumption of Omega 6 fatty acids, especially if not properly balanced with an increased consumption of Omega 3 fatty acids, can irritate the gut lining. A diet rich in Omega 6 fatty acids, such as fried or oily foods, will be more likely to cause such symptoms.

Intestinal Bacteria

As bacteria can access the diverticula pouches and cause infection, it is necessary to understand how to reduce the chances of this happening as well as defining the culprits.

The gut is home to trillions of bacteria. Our gut is inhabited by a collective group of good and bad bacteria, otherwise known as our gut flora or microbiota/microbiome. Our gut microbiome contributes tremendously to our everyday lives, unbeknownst to many. They protect us from organisms that attack our intestines[13],[14]; they assist in the absorption of nutrients and energy from the food we eat[15],[16] (even foods that our body is unable to digest alone); and they help our immune system work at full capacity[17]. In fact, tests that study the effect of probiotic bacteria and antibiotic drugs suggest that the microbiome regulates anxiety, mood, cognition and pain[18]. A bacterial overgrowth observed in patients with Diverticulosis or an unbalanced bacterial ecosystem, has been linked to intestinal inflammation.

If you have previously taken a large dose of antibiotics it is important to take the necessary steps to increase the amounts of good bacteria and achieve symbiosis.

Symptoms Associated with Diverticulitis

There are varying degrees of symptoms in patients with diverticular disease. A frequent symptom is pain that switches on and off in the stomach, often in the lower left-hand side for western people. Shortly after or during a meal this pain often worsens. Passing stools may relieve the pain. Other symptoms include[5]:

- Constipation, diarrhea or periods of constipation followed by diarrhea
- Bloating
- Bleeding from the rectum

Once Diverticulosis has advanced into its more severe stage of Diverticulitis, the pain becomes noticeably more severe and constant. The pain starts below the belly button and moves to the lower left-hand side of the abdomen. Asian people often develop it in the right-hand side. Other symptoms include:

- High temperatures of and exceeding 38 degrees Celsius or 100 degrees Fahrenheit
- Feeling or being sick
- Constipation
- Bleeding from the rectum
- Frequent urination

- Difficulty or pain while urinating

Diagnosing Diverticulitis

Diverticular disease is a tricky condition to diagnose from symptoms alone. However, if anyone experiences the symptoms previously mentioned, it is important to see a doctor immediately.

It is difficult to successfully diagnose Diverticulitis at first glance as it shares similar symptoms with other digestive disorders. When seeing a doctor, it is likely that they will run a series of tests to rule out easily identifiable diseases. A blood test will likely be recommended to rule out coeliac disease. Urine tests will allow signs of infection to be checked. Pregnancy tests may be suggested to women of childbearing age to negate pregnancy as the cause of abdominal pain. Liver function tests negate the possibility of abdominal pain caused by conditions such as alcohol-related liver disease. A stool test may be taken from those that are experiencing diarrhea in order to rule out further infections.

There are a variety of tests a doctor can run if he/she suspects that the symptoms match with digestive disorders such as Diverticulosis[5].

Colonoscopy

When symptoms align with Diverticulosis or Diverticulitis a doctor may advise a colonoscopy. A colonoscopy is the easiest way of looking directly inside the large intestine to check for any bulges or pouches that look like diverticula. During a colonoscopy, a colonoscope is placed into the rectum and further into the colon that houses the pain. A colonoscope is a thin tube that has a camera attached to the end. Laxatives are prescribed beforehand to empty the bowels and allow for an easier diagnosis. Although this sounds extremely uncomfortable, the procedure isn't normally painful. However, you may be given a sedative or painkilling medication beforehand to reduce the uncomfortable feeling and help you feel more at ease.

Barium enema X-ray

Barium is a special liquid; it is used to cover the colon to make it easier to see in X-rays. Barium is special as it coats the inside of organs, allowing hidden parts of organs such as the colon to be displayed. This allows a doctor to investigate how the colon looks and if there are any visible bulges or pouches. Firstly, a laxative will be provided to clear out the colon. A tube will then be inserted into the rectum, squirting the barium into the tube and up through the rectum. A few X-rays will then be taken. Do not worry if stool appears white or discolored for a few days afterwards, this is just the barium safely leaving your body.

CT scans

If you have previous history of diverticular disease or a blood test has shown an unusually high number of white blood cells (which indicated infection) and your symptoms match those of Diverticulitis, a doctor may assume this is the case.

However, a CT scan may be used to rule out other conditions such as gallstones or a hernia. CT or computerized tomography scans take a series of X-rays which are displayed on a computer to build a 3-D image. CT scans are beneficial as they allow large areas to be visualized, which is particularly useful when infections have spread. This may be the case in complications such as abscesses.

How to Prevent Diverticulitis and its Attacks

Unfortunately, there is no known cure for Diverticulosis or Diverticulitis. However, there are some preventative measures that can be taken to reduce the chance of Diverticulitis and Diverticulitis-based attacks from happening. Since over 50% of people aged 80 and older are likely to suffer from Diverticulosis, the following actions should be considered as safety precautions. It's better to be safe than sorry.

Fiber & Diet

A low-fiber diet is widely considered to be the triggering factor behind Diverticulosis. As previously explained, it is thought that consistent hard stools or straining during bowel movements contribute to forming diverticula. If a diet consists of low amounts of fiber, then stools will become harder and more difficult to pass. Therefore, it is recommended to increase the amount of fiber intake, either through diet or supplements[19]. 20 to 38 grams of fiber is recommended each day to prevent Diverticulosis[19]. The second half of this book contains many recipes full containing large fiber contents, as this is the leading hypothesis on the cause of diverticular disease.

Foods rich in fiber include fresh fruits and vegetables, wheat bran, beans and brown or wholegrain rice, etc. If you are struggling to include enough fiber, another tactic is to include foods of liquid consistency such as soups or vegetable-based juices to soften the consistency of stools. Strong evidence shows that insoluble fiber found in fruits and vegetables decrease risk of diverticular disease more effectively than their soluble counterpart. There is also some evidence indicating that the consumption of red meat increases the risk of diverticular disease. As of now, alcohol, caffeine and smoking are known to irritate the digestive system, but in moderation, don't conclusively appear to influence diverticular disease[20].

Eliminate straining

Straining causes undue pressure on the intestines. Sometimes we aren't even aware when it's happening but it's important to be mindful during bowel movements. Even a small amount of straining over a long period of time is enough to weaken the intestines. A high fiber diet reduces the need to strain.

Restore intestinal flora

As mentioned previously, an unbalanced gut flora (dysbiosis) may also contribute to Diverticulitis. The gut flora assists the body in a variety of different manners; including improving mood and the immune system. By restoring balance in the intestinal flora, it'll allow the digestive function to operate normally as well as improve overall health. This is particularly important if you have digested strong antibiotics recently as they kill both good and bad bacteria in a non-selective manner. To remedy this, take probiotics and prebiotics. Probiotics are a collection of live bacteria that can be found in yogurt and other dairy products, while prebiotics are a specialized plant fiber that good bacteria consume to fuel themselves[21].

Reducing intestinal inflammation

The best way to reduce both intestinal inflammation and the chances of causing diverticula is by monitoring your diet. NSAIDs such as ibuprofen are known to cause inflammation[22],[23]. Instead, consume Omega 9 fatty acids, found in foods such as olives and avocados, Omega 3 fatty acids in fish, garlic, herbs such as basil, oregano, parsley and turmeric, and green tea. All these foods are found to reduce inflammation and have the additional effect of improving overall wellbeing.

Eliminate stress

Stress can be defined as a small disruption to the physiological balance. Stress continuously weakens the body, especially the gut[24]. The first recorded observation of stress directly effecting intestinal functions being in 1825 by William Beaumont[25]. He observed an injured soldier with a gastric fistula (a wound in the digestive tract allowing gastric fluids to leak through the stomach lining or intestines) that when the soldier experienced fear or anger, it had a direct impact on his gastric functions, most notably acid secretion.

Stress causes many physiological changes to happen in the body, the most well documented being the release of adrenaline and cortisol hormones by the adrenal glands. These have very important functions in stressful situations. Adrenaline is the fight-or-flight hormone that increases heartrate and breathing, shrinks blood vessels, causes sweating and slows insulin production (insulin is a hormone that allows your body to use glucose found in carbohydrates and sugar into energy). Prolonged exposure to stressful situations & the adrenaline that ensues can cause damaged blood vessels, high blood pressure, headaches, anxiety, insomnia and weight gain. Cortisol increases the amount of glucose in the bloodstream and helps the brain to use it more effectively, increases tissue repair substances, reduces nonessential bodily functions, alters the immune system and dampens the reproductive and growth systems. However, prolonged exposure to cortisol causes weight gain, high blood pressure, sleep problems, lack of energy, type 2 diabetes, osteoporosis, mental cloudiness, memory problems and a weakened immune system.

It's easy to acknowledge when you're stressed but it's harder to act on it. Most people take stress as a necessity, whether it's caused by work, family or just everyday life. There are simple ways to control and reduce stress in a world that is uncontrollable. If you are experiencing consistently high levels of stress, you may want to approach a psychologist for advice. Regular exercise, meditation, breathing techniques or even a 10-minute walk outdoors can help to reduce stress.

Supplements

Preventing Diverticulitis can require a lifestyle change and a lot of effort. There are a vast number of supplements that allow us to meet certain requirements that may be otherwise hard to manage. Below is a list of supplements and the areas they benefit:

Fiber:

- Psyllium Husk Capsules
- Fruit Cubes
- Fiber Capsules
- Partially Hydrolyzed Guar Gum

Intestinal Flora:

- Acidophilus
- Probiotics that include Escherichia Coli strain Nissle 1917 or Probiotics in general
- Prebiotics

Inflammation:

- Omega 3 or Fish Oil Capsules
- Vitamin C Tablets
- Vitamin E Tablets
- Bioflavanoids found in things such as Grape Seed Extract or Garlic Capsules. They are also found in

onions and apples
- Garlic capsules
- Co-enzyme Q10
- Milk Thistle to reduce inflammation in the liver if needed

Surgeries to Remove Diverticulitis

Previously, surgeries were offered to those that had suffered from two or more Diverticulitis attacks as a provision to protect against future attacks and complications. This has changed recently as the general consensus is that the cost outweigh the benefit; an estimated 1 in 100 suffer from complications after surgery[5]. Although there are exceptions where the opposite is true. If you have reoccurring complications or if you have suffered from Diverticulitis at a young age, it may be beneficial to have the surgery, since the longer someone lives with this disease, the higher the chances of complications. There are two main types of surgery associated with Diverticulitis.

Stoma Surgery

In situations where the large intestine is severely damaged, it is recommended that the intestine heal for a minimum of nine weeks to fully recover. This is where stoma surgery is used. A stoma is a small hole in the abdomen that allows waste to pass out into a man-made pouch, bypassing the intestine altogether. There are two types of stoma surgeries.

Ileostomy – The stoma is situated in the stomach. The large intestine is isolated from the small intestine and sealed, allowing adequate time to heal. The small intestine is diverted and joined to the stoma.

Colostomy – Instead of isolating the large intestine, only a small section is isolated. The rest of the large intestine is joined to the stoma in the lower abdomen.

Colectomy

This method involves removing the troublesome part of the large intestine. This may be performed in two ways: an open colectomy or a laparoscopic colectomy. An open colectomy involves the removal of a section of the large intestine through a large incision in the abdomen, while the laparoscopic colectomy is a type of keyhole surgery. This surgery has a good rate of success as an estimated 1 in 12 people having a recurrence of symptoms afterwards[5].

Recent Advancements in Science

Science progresses daily, so much so that it is hard for general practitioners to keep up to date. It's important to note that new information doesn't automatically qualify it as superior information. In fact, studies that have plenty of counterarguments or are used as a basis for further investigation are the most reliable. Although, it never hurts to stay one step ahead. This section summarizes interesting advancements that have occurred in the last few years.

Diagnosis

Discussions of correctly diagnosing diverticular disease are common in recent literature. The first topic relates to differentiating IBS from diverticular disease[26]. This counter-study was originally conducted to investigate claims that people suffering from acute diverticulitis are susceptible to IBS going forwards[27]. This is particularly interesting as both diseases share common symptoms, which is why it's important that medical practitioners have the tools to distinguish between the two. The study concludes that 12.8% of acute diverticulitis patients contacted continued to have diverticular related symptoms, and not solely IBS as the previous study claimed.

A study of 72 patients between 2012 and 2013 was set out to discover the single most characterizing symptom of uncomplicated diverticular disease[28]. Interestingly, this study also made the distinction between IBS and diverticular disease, stating that by definition, IBS is a disease with no structural or organic lesions. The study concluded that "moderate to severe and prolonged left lower-abdominal pain" is the best identifier of diverticular disease.

Treatments

There is not much information on how probiotics affect diverticular disease but an investigation in 2016 aimed in kick-starting it[29]. Unfortunately, this study didn't lead to significant evidence swaying either way, but this is an interesting direction to look at in the future.

11%-38% of people that receive endoscopic treatment for diverticular bleeding are re-admitted into the hospital within 30 days[30]. This next study investigated how high-dose barium impaction; barium that is retained after a barium enema x-ray may actually help to lower the risk of recurrent bleeding[31]. Although the outcome of this study was successful, it requires many more studies with much larger sample sizes to be credible.

Finally, and the most interesting evolution. There has been recent development in the technology used to surgically intervene with those from suffering particularly bad diverticular lesions[32]. A special 'over-the-scope clip' can be attached to endoscopes, allowing the surgeon to enter the intestines and insert a clip, closing the lesion, in one minimally invasive procedure.

Ingredient Analysis

As with many disorders of the gut, diet plays a crucial role in the prevention and healing of this disease. Dietary recommendations differ substantially depending on what stage of this disease the patient is currently experiencing. The two different stages can be defined as; during a flare-up and outside of a flare-up.

During a Flare-Up Diet

This cannot be stressed enough and is the cause of confusion for many people. The recommended diet for someone experiencing acute pain or a flare-up is a short-term liquid diet followed by a low-fiber diet. Once the low-fiber diet can be tolerated, the patient should slowly increase their fiber until eating a regular healthy diet. For detailed information on the recommended liquid diet or low-fiber diet during those stages of Diverticulitis, please visit the chapter: "Diet During A Flare Up or Acute Pain" in the "Recipes" section. If you are suffering from pain, take immediate advice from your doctor. It is extremely important to get professional help if; your abdominal pain increases over time, you're unable consume clear liquids without vomiting or if you develop a fever.

Ingredients for the General Prevention of Diverticulitis

The earlier chapter "How to Prevent Diverticulitis and its Attacks" states that there are three main targets that a prevention diet should aim for, these are; increasing fiber, increasing the variety of intestinal flora and reducing intestinal inflammation.

By taking a logical approach, we can analyze which molecules, vitamins and minerals positively and negatively affect each of the three goals. It's then a matter of finding a combination of ingredients, once combined, that not only create a delicious recipe but actively work towards one or more of these goals. For example, a mixture of fruit (with its skin left on) and Greek yoghurt creates an easy breakfast that is high in fiber (due to the fruit), increases intestinal flora count (due to Greek yoghurt) and also provides prebiotics to feed the good gut bacteria (from the fruit skin). You are welcome to mix and match any of the ingredients from the categories to your heart's, or palette's, content. Since costs of products vary per country, per region and per shop, the cost category is a rough estimation of how that food compares to other foods within that category. The cheapest being $ and most expensive being $$$. For example, the cheapest no-thrills pack of old-fashioned oats can be purchased for around $0.09 per ounce or $0.31 per 100 grams. Whereas buckwheat can cost $0.44 per ounce or $1.55 per 100 grams.

High Fiber Foods

As mentioned previously, it is recommended to consume 20 to 38 grams of fiber per day to prevent Diverticulosis[19]. It is also widely considered that a low fiber intake is one of the leading causes of diverticular disease, as a moderate intake in fiber helps to create healthy stool. Meat and processed foods have either 0 grams of fiber or extremely small amounts.

Grains

As a general rule, all grains, especially wholegrains, are high in fiber. Wholegrain simply means that the entirety of the grain is left intact, essentially the grain is left as it was growing in the field. Advancement in milling technology allowed the bran and germ to be removed cheaply and easily, turning wholegrains such as brown rice into a refined version, white rice. The center part of the grain, endosperm, is considered the most flavorful and is easier to cook than the wholegrain. However, we are now aware that roughly 70% of the nutrients come from the other two parts of the grain, the bran and germ. There is also a lot more fiber in wholegrain than refined grain, for example, whole wheat flour contains roughly 4-5x more fiber than white flour.

High Fiber Grains

Food	Fiber per cup	Fiber per 100 grams	Cost
Oats	16.5	10.6	$
Buckwheat	17	10	$$
Wholegrain Cornmeal	8.9	7.3	$
Whole-wheat Bread (per slice)	1.9	6	$
Bulgur	8.2	4.5	$
Whole-wheat Pasta	4.5	3.9	$
Quinoa	5.2	2.8	$$

Food	Fiber per cup	Fiber per 100 grams	Cost
Brown Rice	3.5	1.8	$
Couscous	2.2	1.4	$$
Egg Noodles	1.9	1.2	$
Rice Noodles	1.8	1	$

Low Fiber Grains for Comparison

Food	Fiber per cup	Fiber per 100 grams
White Pasta	3.7	3.2
White Bread	0.8 per slice	2.7
White Rice	0.6	0.4

Fruits

If the skin of the fruit is kept on, most fruits are high in fiber. Prices for the same fruit vary depending on the season. Not only is it much cheaper to buy berries frozen, the fiber content is often nearly identical, making frozen berries a good option for a snackable smoothie. Avoid all fruit juices that do not contain pulp as this is where the vast majority of the fiber resides.

Food	Fiber per medium fruit or cup if stated	Fiber per 100 grams	Cost

Food	Fiber per medium fruit or cup if stated	Fiber per 100 grams	Cost
Avocado	13.5	6.7	$$$
Raspberries	8 per cup	6.5	$$
Blackberries	7.6 per cup	5.3	$
Dried Cranberries	4 per cup	5.3	$$
Pomegranate	11.3	4	$$
Pears	5.5	3.1	$
Dried Fig	1.5	2.9	$$
Bananas	3.1	2.6	$
Oranges	3.1	2.4	$
Blueberries	3.6 per cup	2.4	$
Red Delicious Apples	4.9	2.3	$
Strawberries	3.3 per cup	2	$

Vegetables

As a general rule, the darker vegetables contain more fiber. As with fruit, do not remove the skin to optimize fiber intake. Vegetables that are mostly comprised of water such as iceberg lettuce and any vegetables that have been overcooked contain low amounts of fiber.

Food	Fiber per cup	Fiber per 100 grams	Cost
Artichoke	7.7	5.4	$$

Parsnips	6.5	4.9	$
Collards	1.4	4	$
Brussel Sprouts	4.1	3.8	$
Kale	2.6	3.6	$
Broccoli	5.1	3.3	$
Sweet Potatoes	6.6	3.3	$
Butternut squash	6.6	3.2	$
Carrots	4.7	3	$
Eggplant	2.5	3	$
Asparagus	2.8	2.1	$$
Beets	3.4	2	$
Leeks	1.6	1.8	$

Legumes

Legumes price vary dramatically depending on whether you buy them as dried beans or canned. If dried, they often require a lot of preparation before cooking. Some dried beans require 10 hours of soaking plus an additional few hours of simmering before being edible. You can buy dried beans in larger quantities since they often grow tremendously in size after being exposed to water, such as dried chickpeas tripling in size after being soaked and boiled. Since the dried beans and canned beans vary in price so significantly, there will not be a cost category in this section. Please note, most recipes in this book state that the legumes come from a can, as they are precooked and are much easier to cook with.

Food	Fiber per cup	Fiber per 100 grams
White Beans	18.6	10.4
Kidney Beans	16.5	9.3
Pinto Beans	15.4	9
Black Beans	15	8.7
Split Peas	16.3	8.3
Lentils	15.6	7.9
Chickpeas	12.5	7.6
Black-eyed Peas	11.1	6.5
Peas	8.3	5.7
Baked Beans	13.9	5.5
Lima Beans	9.2	5.4
Refried Beans	11.4	4.7

Nuts & Seeds

Nuts and seeds are overwhelmingly fibrous and packed with nutrients. They are also high in calories and Omega 6, which can cause inflammation if not balanced with Omega 3. As with everything, moderation is key. First theorized in 1958, diverticulitis advice from the medical community discouraged patients from consuming seeds, as it was thought that seeds can become trapped in diverticular pouches. Recent studies have debunked this claim, particularly since there has been no clinical evidence since 1958, but also as one large study showed that the consumption of seeds and nuts had a positive effect on reducing diverticulitis onset[2].

Food	Fiber per cup	Fiber per 100 grams	Cost
Chia Seeds	9.8	34.4	$$
Flax Seeds	7.8	27.3	$$$
Almonds	3.6	12.5	$$
Sunflower Seeds	3.2	11.1	$
Pistachios	3	10.6	$$$
Hazelnuts	2.8	9.7	$$$
Pecans	2.7	9.6	$$$
Dry Roasted Peanuts	2.4	9.4	$
Brazil Nuts	2.1	7.5	$$$
Walnuts	5.4	6.7	$$$

Intestinal Flora Diversification

A highly diverse intestinal flora contributes to general digestive wellbeing & assists with all manners of digestion[13,15]. There are two main methods for increasing intestinal flora count;

consuming foods rich with live bacteria and yeasts (aka probiotics) or consuming foods that gut microflora consume themselves (aka prebiotics) such as the fibrous foods mentioned above or foods rich with molecules that allow healthy bacteria to flourish.

Probiotics

It is difficult to produce probiotic rich food as bacteria need to live in specific states to survive and grow. Fermentation is the process of allowing bacteria or yeast to breakdown carbohydrates over a period of time, allowing the bacteria to multiply. Even if a product is fermented, applying moderate amounts of heat to the product can kill off healthy bacteria.

Probiotic-rich Foods

Food	Description	Cost
Kefir	Kefir is a fermented probiotic drink that is produced by adding cultures of bacteria and yeast to goat or cow's milk. It is one of the best sources of probiotics.	$
Live Yogurts such as Greek or Probiotic Yogurt	It is important to check labelling to make sure your yoghurt contains live or active cultures. Bacteria is easily killed off and the manufacturer will have to produce the yoghurt with as little heat as possible. Try to avoid artificially sweetened yogurts.	$
Miso Soup or Paste	A Japanese seasoning made from fermenting soybeans with salt and a type of fungus.	$

Food	Description	Cost
Tempeh	Another fermented soybean that consists of a nutty, firm patty. The fermentation process adds vitamin B12 which soybeans do not naturally contain as its mainly found in meat, fish and dairy. Tempeh is a great choice for vegetarians.	$$
Traditional Buttermilk	Buttermilk can be misleading. There are two types, traditional and cultured. Traditional buttermilk is the leftover liquid from making butter and is mainly consumed in India, Nepal & Pakistan. This type of buttermilk contains a good source of probiotics. Cultured buttermilk is fermented pasteurized low-fat or nonfat milk. The pasteurization process kills of the good bacteria. Cultured buttermilk found in American supermarkets do not contain probiotics.	$$$
Sauerkraut	Sauerkraut is fermented cabbage. The taste can vary dramatically depending on the producer but is defined by its sour & salty taste. Only buy unpasteurized sauerkraut as pasteurization kills live bacteria.	$
Kimchi	Kimchi is a mixture of fermented cabbage, chili flakes and other vegetables such as garlic and scallion. It is normally eaten as a side dish in Korea or fried together with rice.	$$

Food	Description	Cost
Kombucha	Kombucha is a fermented black or green tea drink. However, high heat is known to kill bacteria and there's a lack of high-quality evidence on the probiotic benefits of kombucha.	$$
Pickles	Pickles that are created from pickled cucumber in salt and water contain healthy probiotics. Cucumbers pickled in vinegar do not contain probiotics.	$
Gouda, Mozzarella, Cheddar & Cottage Cheese	It is important to look for live or active cultures on the food labels of cheese before buying it. Not all cheese contains probiotics.	$$
Red Wine	Alcohol is highly toxic and any form of excess alcohol damages the gut. However, due to the high number of polyphenols contained in red wine, it's been observed that low to moderate consumption increased healthy bacteria and decreased harmful bacteria. Avoiding alcohol altogether is the best option, but if you have to choose, red wine is the only type of alcohol with positive effects.	$$

Probiotic-harming Foods

Food	Description
Alcohol	All excessive forms of alcohol have been observed to be harmful to the gut microbiome.
Artificial Sweeteners	Artificial sweetener fed mice have been observed to have a reduction in positive gut bacteria. The research is in its early stages and the same results haven't been consistently observed in humans. It appears that consuming artificial sweeteners over sugar has some negative effects in some people, and no effects in others. More research is needed.

Prebiotics

Prebiotics refer to the dietary fiber that feeds healthy bacteria, helping them to survive and grow. Some types of Dietary Fibers include Inulin, Fructooligosaccharides (FOS), Beta-glucan, Arabinoxylan Oligosaccharides (AXOS) and Galacto-oligosaccharides (GOS)[33]. Fibrous vegetables are a great source of prebiotics alongside select fruits. Foods without dietary fiber, such as processed snacks, meat or dairy contain limited or zero prebiotic benefits.

Food	Prebiotic Fiber	Cost
Sunchokes aka Jerusalem Artichokes	Inulin and FOS	$$
Garlic	Inulin and FOS	$

Food	Prebiotic Fiber	Cost
Onions	Inulin and FOS	$
Leeks	Inulin and FOS	$
Asparagus	Inulin and FOS	$$
Bananas	Inulin and FOS	$
Sweet Potatoes	Inulin and FOS	$$$
Oats	Beta-glucan	$
Wheat Bran	AXOS	$
Apples	Pectin, Sorbitol & Mannitol	$
Flaxseed	Mucilage & Lignin	$$$
Beans and Peas	GOS	$

Reducing Inflammation

Inflammation can rupture diverticulum causing diverticulitis. For those suffering with diverticulosis, it's possible to significantly reduce the chances of suffering with major complications and continue to live a normal life by reducing inflammation. Similarly, those currently suffering with diverticulitis can reduce the chances of having a diverticulitis attack by following the same advice.

It's important to note that Omega 6 fatty acids are healthy for the human body so long as they are balanced with Omega 3 fatty acids[34]. Our modern diet has evolved to include more meat and fried food and less fish, resulting in the diet of an average western citizen being a ratio of 1:15 of Omega 3 fatty acids to Omega 6 fatty acids (for every 15 grams of Omega 6 consumed, only 1 gram of Omega 3 is consumed), whereas the recommended balance is 1:4 (or 0.25:1). To-date there is no scientific consensus on how Omega 6s are pro-inflammatory. A study in 2012 by the Journal of Nutrition and Metabolism suggests that the anti-inflammatory benefits of Omega 3 have been seen to be cancelled out by an abundance of Omega 6, therefore it is an oversimplification to state that Omega 6 is inherently pro-inflammatory but an abundance of Omega 6 is potentially harmful nonetheless[34].

For the purpose of this section, beneficial anti-inflammatory foods will include those with a ratio of Omega 3 to Omega 6 of 1:4 or higher. However, do not purposely remove Omega 6 completely from your diet, as with everything, moderation is key.

Anti-Inflammatory Foods

Omega 3 Fatty Acids (Omega 3 to Omega 6 Ratio =>1:4)

By and large, the best source of Omega 3 is oily fish. Although there are no uniform standards for daily recommended Omega 3 intake, the Food and Nutrition Board of the US Institute of Medicine recommend 1.6 grams for men and 1.1 grams for women aged 19 years and older[35].

Food	Grams of Omega 3 Per Ounce	Grams of Omega 3 Per 100g	Omega 3: Omega 6 Ratio	Cost

Food	Grams of Omega 3 Per Ounce	Grams of Omega 3 Per 100g	Omega 3: Omega 6 Ratio	Cost
Bluefin Tuna	0.4	1.7	25:1	$$
Cod Liver Oil	5.5	19.7	21:1	$$
Anchovies	0.4	1.5	16:1	$$
Pacific Herring	0.7	2.6	14:1	$$
Atlantic Mackerel	0.3	1.3	12:1	$$
Flaxseeds	6.4	22	3:1	$$
Flaxseed Oil	15	53	3:1	$$
Chia Seeds	5	17.8	3:1	$$
Canned Sardines	0.3	1.1	3:1	$
Atlantic Salmon	0.7	2.5	3:1	$$
Walnuts	2.5	9	1:4	$$$

Omega 9 Fatty Acids

Omega 3 and Omega 6 are "essential fats", which means the body can't naturally produce them and they must be obtained entirely through diet. On the other hand, Omega 9 is non-essential, meaning that it is naturally produced by the body. Some studies have found that consuming Omega 9 had anti-inflammatory benefits in both mice and humans[36].

Food	Grams of Omega 9	Cost

Food	Per Ounce	Per 100g	Cost
Almonds	30	105	$$
Cashews	24	84	$$
Olive Oil	23	83	$
Almond Oil	19	70	$$$
Avocado Oil	17	60	$$
Peanut Oil	13	47	$
Walnuts	9	31	$$$

Pro-Inflammatory Foods

Omega 6 Fatty Acids (Omega 3 to Omega 6 Ratio <1:4)

As stated earlier, Omega 6 isn't inherently bad as long as it's balanced adequately with the consumption of Omega 3. Please note, there are various nut-based oils that contains no Omega 3, denoted by the "Omega 3: Omega 6 Ratio" column being "N/A". Although cheap, these oils should be avoided. Some nuts and seeds contain a large amount of Omega 6, making portion control important. One medium handful of almonds, or roughly 20 grams, would equate to 2.4 grams of Omega 6.

Food	Grams of Omega 6 Per Ounce	Grams of Omega 6 Per 100g	Omega 3: Omega 6 Ratio	Cost
Grapeseed Oil	19	69	N/A	$
Peanut Oil	9	32	N/A	$
Sunflower Seeds	6.5	23	N/A	$

Food	Grams of Omega 6 Per Ounce	Grams of Omega 6 Per 100g	Omega 3: Omega 6 Ratio	Cost
Almond Oil	4.9	17	N/A	$$$
Almonds	3.4	12	1:4109	$$
Cashews	2.2	7.7	1:125	$$
Corn Oil	15	53	1:46	$
KFC Fried Chicken Breast	1.6	0.2	1:20	$$$
Cured Ham	0.4	1.6	1:10	$$$
Nachos with Cheese	1.2	4.4	1:7	$
Firm Tofu	1.2	0.5	1:7	$

The Most Beneficial Foods

Cover Multiple Categories

Flaxseeds and Walnuts are the star of the show. One tablespoon of Flaxseeds added to a yoghurt or smoothie adds an additional 11% of your daily recommended Fiber, which is also a great source of Mucilage and Lignin Prebiotics as well as providing an astounding 2.3 grams of Omega 3 fatty acids, which is 0.7 higher than the recommended daily intake for men and 1.2 higher than for women. 1 ounce (28g) of Walnuts are 8% of your daily recommended Fiber, 2.5 grams of Omega 3,

10 grams of Omega 6 (making the ratio 1:4) and 9 grams of Omega 9, making them the only nut to contain a significant amount of the anti-inflammatory Omega 3 alpha-linolenic acid (ALA).

Food	Category
Flax Seeds	Fiber, Prebiotic & Omega 3
Walnuts	Fiber, Omega 3 & Omega 9
Almonds	Fiber & Omega 9
Chia Seeds	Fiber & Omega 3
Beans & Peas	Fiber & Prebiotic
Bananas	Fiber & Prebiotic
Oats	Fiber & Prebiotic
Sweet Potatoes	Fiber & Prebiotic

Bang for your Buck

Nuts, fish or fruit and vegetables that aren't in season are generally more expensive than their processed food counterparts. However, there are certain foods that stand out as being the cheapest in their category whilst simultaneously providing a similar amount of nutrients. Flax seeds and chia seeds are kept on this list since they provide multiple benefits, meaning multiple times the value per dollar.

Food	Category

Food	Category
Flax Seeds	Fiber, Prebiotic & Omega 3
Oats	Fiber & Prebiotic
Bananas	Fiber & Prebiotic
Chia Seeds	Fiber & Prebiotic
Wholegrain Bread	Fiber
Greek Yoghurt	Probiotics
Sauerkraut	Probiotics
Canned Sardines	Omega 3
Olive Oil	Omega 9

The Most Harmful Foods

Unsurprisingly the most harmful foods are also the most processed. Chocolate bars, candies and sugary breakfast cereals can contribute to intestinal inflammation. Fast food is often fried in a lot of cheap oils, providing an excess of Omega 6 which then becomes pro-inflammatory. Red meat is not a sufficient source of fiber, prebiotics, probiotics, Omega 3 or Omega 9. Therefore, red meat consumption can be minimized with the savings going towards more beneficial types of food. However, red meat is not harmful in moderation unless heavily fried.

Help Shape Our Books

If this book has helped you at all, I'd love to read your feedback on Amazon. You can leave a review by following this link or going directly to Amazon: https://bit.ly/3hMZ8Mj. Reviews help us refine our books, making our next one that little bit more helpful.

If you'd like to stay up-to-date with our publications, or would just like to drop us a message, feel free to email us at info.healthful@gmail.com. You can also follow us on www.facebook.com/healthfulpublications. Thanks for reading so far and we hope you enjoy the recipes!

Recipes

During A Flare-Up or Acute Pain

First and foremost, if you are suffering from pain, take immediate advice from your doctor. It is extremely important to get professional help if; your abdominal pain increases over time, you're unable consume clear liquids without vomiting or if you develop a fever. These symptoms may indicate the need for hospitalization. Physicians commonly recommend a liquid based diet until the pain subsides. A liquid diet relieves pressure from your gut, giving it time to rest until any diarrhea or bleeding reduces. The diet should only be maintained for a few days, otherwise you will miss out essential nutrients and vitamins from solid food sources. Initially, clear liquids such as the following should be consumed:

- Clear broth without solid food
- Fruit juices without pulp
- Ice lollipops without fruit pulp
- Gelatin
- Water
- Tea or coffee without cream (in moderation)

Once the pain starts to diminish and you start to feel better, you should slowly start consuming low-fiber foods such as:

- Canned or cooked fruits without skin or seeds

- Canned or cooked vegetables such as green beans, carrots and potatoes (without the skin)
- Eggs, fish and poultry
- Refined white bread
- Fruit and vegetable juice with no pulp
- Low-fiber cereals
- Milk, yogurt and cheese
- White rice, pasta and noodles

This is a short-term diet recommended to transition through diverticular pain. Once this low-fiber diet is tolerable, you can slowly increase fiber intake until capable of consuming a normal diet.

A study published in 2017 explored the effects of continuing a normal diet instead of the recommended approach above whilst patients are experiencing a flare-up[37]. Unfortunately, 19.8% of patients experienced continuing symptoms 6 months after their flare-up. Therefore, it is recommended to follow a specific strategy during both stages of the flare-up. Because of this reason, this book does not provide any recipes during this stage as it is critical to follow your physician's bespoke advice.

Diverticulitis Prevention Diet

This section takes all of the most beneficial ingredients from the previous section and suggests recipes for breakfast, lunch and dinner. They are broken down, explaining exactly why they are beneficial, their macronutrients and their estimated value. The macronutrients are taken from U.S.

Department of Agriculture, Agricultural Research Service, FoodData Central, fdc.nal.usda.gov. All recipes contain both US Imperial and Metric measurements for readers all around the world.

Please note, the value calculation is a rough estimate as prices for ingredients vary depending on the season, the location and the producer. There is also a differentiation between the total cost of a meal's ingredients and the price per macronutrients. For example, Flax seeds can be quite expensive, but they provide fiber, prebiotics and Omega 3. Therefore, the money spent on flax seeds provides 3x the benefit as the money spent on oats.

Breakfast

Crunchy Fruit Pot

Macronutrients & Omegas per Serving

Kcal:	486	**Carbs:**	68.3g	**Omega 3:**	2.4g
Fat:	15.2g	**Fiber:**	13.3g	**Omega 6:**	2g
Protein:	24g	**Cholesterol:**	20mg	**Ratio:**	1.21:1

Boasting a high amount of fiber and prebiotics from Oats and Fruit, a source of Probiotics from Yoghurt and Anti-Inflammatory Omega 3s and Omega 9s from flax seeds. If adding additional fruit, make sure to leave the skin on to keep all the fiber and prebiotics. Flax seeds can be switched with chia seeds for a cheaper alternative.

Benefits: Fiber, Prebiotics, Probiotics & Anti-Inflammatory
Value: $$
Time: 5 mins
Serves: 1
Ingredients
1 Banana
1/3 Cup (50g) Raspberries
1/4 Cup (40g) Oats
3/4 Cup (150g) Greek Yoghurt
1 Tbsp Flax seed

Method
1. Mix the flax seeds, oats and Greek yoghurt in a bowl.

2. Slice the banana and add it to the bottom of a separate bowl or wide glass. Top the banana with the yoghurt mixture. Add the berries on top and serve.

Apple & Seed Porridge

Macronutrients & Omegas per Serving

Kcal:	427	**Carbs:**	79.1g	**Omega 3:**	0.1g
Fat:	7.3g	**Fiber:**	9.8g	**Omega 6:**	1.1g
Protein:	11.9g	**Cholesterol:**	13mg	**Ratio:**	0.12:1

A cheap breakfast that will leave you satiated for the whole morning. Both the oats and apple contain fiber and prebiotics to feed your good gut bacteria and allow for easy digestion.

Benefits: Fiber & Prebiotics
Value: $
Time: Less than 10 mins
Serves: 4

Ingredients
4 Red Delicious Apples
1 Cup (160g) Oats
2 1/4 Cups (500ml) Whole Milk
3oz (85g) Sultanas
1 Tsp Ground Cinnamon

Method
1. Core and dice the apples.

2. Add the oats and milk to a small saucepan, bring to boil then simmer for 3 mins, stirring occasionally. Add the sultanas, apples and cinnamon, cooking for an additional 2 mins until the porridge is creamy. Serve hot.

Whole Wheat Banana Bread

Macronutrients & Omegas per Serving

Kcal:	573	**Carbs:**	93.3g	**Omega 3:**	0.2g
Fat:	21.2g	**Fiber:**	8.1g	**Omega 6:**	2.6g
Protein:	10.8g	**Cholesterol:**	82mg	**Ratio:**	0.08:1

A great way to use up any overripe bananas. This delicious bread is full of Fiber & Prebiotics from the Whole Wheat Flour & Bananas.

Benefits: Fiber, Prebiotics & Anti-Inflammatory
Value: $
Time: 1 Hour 45 mins
Serves: 4

Ingredients
2 Eggs
3 Mashed Banana
1/4 Cup (60ml) Hot Water
1/2 Cup (170g) Honey
1 3/4 Cups (210g) Whole Wheat Flour
1/2 Tsp Salt
1/2 Tsp Cinnamon, Plus More for Topping
1 Tsp Vanilla Extract
1 Tsp Baking Soda
5 Tbsp Olive Oil

Method

1. Preheat oven to 325°F (165 °C) and grease a 9×5-inch (23x13cm) loaf pan.

2. Add oil, honey, 1/4 cup water & 1tsp baking soda into a large bowl and mix well. After mixing, add the eggs and beat thoroughly.

3. Add the mashed bananas, vanilla, salt and cinnamon into the bowl, stir well. Finally stir in the flour until combined.

4. Pour the batter evenly into the greased loaf pan.

5. Sprinkle with cinnamon, you can use a toothpick or the tip of a butter knife to make a pattern.

6. Bake for 60 mins. Check the bread is done by inserting a toothpick in the top, if it doesn't come out dry bake for an additional 5 mins. Remove from oven and leave it to cool for 5 mins in the pan. Transfer it to a wire rack to cool for 30 minutes before serving.

Note: Recipe adapted from cookieandkate.com

Blackberry, Apple & Pear Oat Bake

Macronutrients & Omegas per Serving

Kcal:	424	**Carbs:**	53.8g	**Omega 3:**	0.3g
Fat:	19.1g	**Fiber:**	11.8g	**Omega 6:**	4.6g
Protein:	13.6g	**Cholesterol:**	38mg	**Ratio:**	0.07:1

A delicious, fruity baked breakfast that can be made ahead of time in batches. Maple syrup will give this breakfast dish a more dessert-like feel. Be sure to use fresh milk as older milk is acidic, and milk curdles if it's heated while acidic.

Benefits: Fiber, Prebiotics & Probiotics
Value: $$
Time: 1 Hour
Serves: 6
Ingredients
1 Egg
2 Red Delicious Apples
2 Pears
6 Cardamom Pods, Bashed or 1/4 Tsp Ground Cardamom
1 Cup (100g) Pecans
1 1/4 Cup (200g) Oats
2 1/4 Cups (320g) Blackberries
17floz (500ml) Fresh Whole Milk
1 Tsp (4g) Ground Cinnamon
1 Tsp Vanilla Extract
1 Tsp Baking Powder
Greek Yogurt to Serve

Method
1. Heat the oven to 400°F (200°C)/350°F (180°C) fan/ gas 6. Core and cut the apples and pears into 0.5-inch (1cm) cubes, chop the pecans and beat the egg.

2. Add the apple, pears, spices and milk into a small saucepan. Cover and gently bring to the boil, simmer for 10 mins. Take off the heat and allow it to infuse for 15 mins minimum.

3. Discard the spice. Pour the mixture into a large bowl and crush the apples and pears with the back of a fork. Mix in the beaten egg, oats, vanilla, baking powder, pecans and blackberries.

4. Pour evenly into a 2-quart (2-liter) ovenproof dish and bake for 30 mins or until the middle is piping hot. Serve with yogurt.

Breakfast Burrito

Macronutrients & Omegas per Serving

Kcal:	416	**Carbs:**	40.7g	**Omega 3:**	0.2g
Fat:	21.8g	**Fiber:**	13g	**Omega 6:**	2.5g
Protein:	14.5g	**Cholesterol:**	166mg	**Ratio:**	0.1:1

Full of healthy fats from the avocado and a little spicy tang from the chipotle paste. This is a perfect dish to make two days in a row to finish off the avocado…although the taste will have you making a second rather quickly.

Benefits: Fiber & Probiotics
Value: $$
Time: 5 mins
Serves: 1

Ingredients
½ Small Avocado, Stoned & Peeled
1 Egg
1 Whole Wheat Tortilla Wrap
7 Cherry Tomatoes (200g)
3 Cups (50g) Kale
1 Tsp (5g) Chipotle Paste
1 Tsp Olive Oil
1 Tbsp Greek Yogurt

Method
1. Halve the cherry tomatoes and slice the avocado. Add the egg, a little salt and pepper as well as the chipotle paste to a bowl. Whisk until the egg is airy.

2. Heat the oil on a medium heat in a large frying pan.

3. Add the kale and tomatoes, cooking until the tomatoes have softened and the kale has reduced in size. Move them to one side of the pan.

4. Pour the egg and chipotle mixture into the empty half of the pan and scramble.

5. Warm the wrap then spoon in Greek yogurt, eggs, kale and tomatoes evenly to the center. Finally, top with avocado and serve.

Smoked Salmon & Tomato Omelet

Macronutrients & Omegas per Serving

Kcal:	225	**Carbs:**	6.9g	**Omega 3:**	0.4g
Fat:	11.8g	**Fiber:**	1.5g	**Omega 6:**	1.8g
Protein:	22.4g	**Cholesterol:**	342mg	**Ratio:**	0.21:1

A high protein meal that's healthy for the brain and gut bacteria. Omelets are versatile, allowing you to add or remove vegetables or meat depending on your goal. The Omega 3 content of the salmon is great for keeping inflammation in check.

Benefits: Probiotics
Value: $$$
Time: 10 mins
Serves: 2

Ingredients
Butter to Grease the Pan
2 Tomatoes (246g)
4 Eggs
3.5oz (100g) Smoked Salmon
1 Tsp Chopped Parsley
1 Tsp Chopped Basil
2 Tbsp (60ml) Whole Milk

Method

1. Add the butter to a non-stick frying pan and warm on medium heat, tilting the pan until the melted butter covers the entire bottom.

2. Beat the eggs & herbs together in a bowl, add a pinch of salt and pepper.

3. Cook the tomatoes for 2 mins until they start to soften. Add the eggs and herb mixture.

4. Stir the eggs gently allowing uncooked egg on the surface of the mixture to fall to the base of the pan between cooked egg. Once there is no visible raw egg, stop stirring and allow the mixture to cook into an omelet.

5. Add the smoked salmon to the center of the omelet and cook for 30 seconds. Cook the omelet to your desired texture.

6. Once finished, slowly tilt the pan and move one side of the omelet to a plate, folding over the farthest side so the salmon is neatly tucked in the middle. Serve immediately.

Apple & Cardamom Quinoa Porridge

Macronutrients & Omegas per Serving

Kcal:	397	**Carbs:**	70.5g	**Omega 3:**	0.1g
Fat:	7.7g	**Fiber:**	8.9g	**Omega 6:**	1.5g
Protein:	12.1g	**Cholesterol:**	13mg	**Ratio:**	0.08:1

A flavorful twist on the classic porridge. The red delicious apples can be switched out for different ripe fruit, just make sure they contain plenty prebiotics. Remove the maple syrup if you prefer a less sweet breakfast.

Benefits: Fiber and Prebiotics
Value: $$
Time: 20 mins
Serves: 2

Ingredients
2 Red Delicious Apples
4 Cardamom Pods
1oz (25g) Oats
2.5oz (75g) Quinoa
8.5floz (250ml) Fresh Whole Milk
1 Tsp Maple Syrup

Method

1. Add 3.5floz (100ml) of milk and 8.5floz (250ml) of water into a small saucepan. Add the cardamom pods, quinoa and oats. Bring to a boil then simmer gently for 15 mins, stirring occasionally to stop the bottom of the pan from burning the quinoa or oats.

2. Pour in the remaining milk and cook for an additional 5 mins until creamy. While cooking, cut the apples into slices.

3. Remove the cardamom pods, pour into bowls and top with the apples and maple syrup.

Overnight Apple & Banana Muesli

Macronutrients & Omegas per Serving

Kcal:	447	**Carbs:**	62.2g	**Omega 3:**	2.1g
Fat:	17.9g	**Fiber:**	9.8g	**Omega 6:**	6.2g
Protein:	13.8g	**Cholesterol:**	7mg	**Ratio:**	0.34:1

A breakfast that requires no cooking and can be made the night before, perfect for preparation for a busy day. Filled to the brim with various Omegas from the nut sources as well as plenty of fiber, prebiotics and probiotics. This crunchy breakfast checks all of the boxes.

Benefits: Fiber, Prebiotics, Probiotics & Anti-Inflammatory
Value: $$$
Time: 5 mins
Serves: 2

Ingredients
1 Red Delicious Apple
1 Banana
1 Walnut
1 Brazil Nut
4 Hazelnuts
1/3 Cup (50g) Oats
1/2 Tsp Ground Cinnamon
2 Tsp Sunflower Seeds
2 Tsp Pumpkin Seeds
1 Tbsp Flax Seeds
3 Tbsp Sultanas
5 1/2 Tbsp Greek Yogurt

Method

1. Chop the brazil nuts, hazelnuts and walnuts. Slice the banana.

2. Grate the red delicious apple into a bowl and add the cinnamon, oats, seeds and half the nuts. Stir together well.

3. Add the yoghurt and 3.5floz (100ml) cold water, stir well and then cover and chill the mixture overnight or for a few hours.

4. When ready to eat, spoon the muesli into 2 bowls, top with the sultanas, banana and remaining nuts.

Strawberry & Avocado Smoothie

Macronutrients & Omegas per Serving

Kcal:	205	**Carbs:**	17.7g	**Omega 3:**	0.2g
Fat:	12.7g	**Fiber:**	4.9g	**Omega 6:**	1.1g
Protein:	7.9g	**Cholesterol:**	15mg	**Ratio:**	0.17:1

A sharp and fruity pick-me-up that can be drank on the commute to work or as an afternoon snack. Smoothies are cheaper than the ready-made alternative, with the added bonus of allowing you to switch out sugar-filled yoghurt to probiotic-filled yogurt.

Benefits: Fiber, Prebiotics and Probiotics
Value: $$$
Time: 5 mins
Serves: 4

Ingredients
Squeeze of Lemon or Lime Juice
1 Avocado, Stoned, Peeled & Cut into Chunks
1/2 Cup (140g) Greek Yogurt
2 Cups (300g) Strawberries
13.5floz (400ml) Whole Milk
1 Tsp (7g) Honey

Method
1. Simply add all the ingredients to a blender and blend until smooth. Add a little water if too thick and blend again.

Nutty Bread with Seeds and Dried Fig served with Cottage Cheese and Apple

Macronutrients & Omegas per Serving

Kcal:	399	**Carbs:**	53.5g	**Omega 3:**	1.4g
Fat:	16.9g	**Fiber:**	8.1g	**Omega 6:**	5.9g
Protein:	13.1g	**Cholesterol:**	24mg	**Ratio:**	0.23:1

This crispy, nutty bread is a supercharged version of whole wheat bread. Containing the regular high dose of fiber that you get with whole wheat bread but pushed to its prebiotics and probiotic limit. This loaf will last in the fridge for 1 month.

Benefits: Fiber, Prebiotics, Probiotics & Anti-Inflammatory
Value: $$$
Time: 1 Hour 30
Serves: 8

Ingredients
1 Large Egg
1 Red Delicious Apple
12 Dried Figs (100g), Thinly Sliced
1/3 Cup (50g) Oats
3/4 Cup (75g) Walnuts
1 1/2 Cups (200g) Self-Raising Whole Wheat Flour
1oz (30g each) Almonds, Brazil Nuts & Hazelnuts
1oz (25g) Cottage Cheese Per Person
5oz (140g) Sultanas
13.5floz (400ml) Hot Black Tea
1 Tsp Baking Powder
1 Tbsp + 2 Tsp (16g) Flax Seeds
3 Tbsp (25g) Pumpkin Seed

Method
1. Heat oven to 350°F (170°C)/300°F (150°C) fan/gas mark 3 1/2.

2. Add the oats, sultanas and figs into a large bowl with the hot tea, stir well and put to one side.

3. Line the base and sides of a 2lb (1kg) loaf tin with baking parchment. Separate 1/2 Cup (50g) of walnuts and the 2 tsp of flax seeds from the rest of the nuts and seeds, these will be used in the topping later. In a bowl add the flour, baking powder and the remaining nuts and seeds that won't be used for topping. Stir well.

4. Beat the egg into the cooled fruity tea mixture, add the flour and seeds mixture and stir well. Pour into the tin, make sure the top is level. Place the rest of the walnuts and flax seeds on top.

5. Bake for 1 hour then cover the top with foil and bake for 15 mins longer. A toothpick inserted into the center of the loaf should come out clean.

6. Remove from the tin, leaving the parchment on until the loaf has cooled, and the parchment is cold.

7. When ready to serve, cut into slices, spread with cottage cheese and slices of apple.

Lunch

Lentil & Sweet Potato Soup

Macronutrients & Omegas per Serving

Kcal:	331	**Carbs:**	54g	**Omega 3:**	0.1g
Fat:	9.2g	**Fiber:**	11.7g	**Omega 6:**	0.8g
Protein:	9.3g	**Cholesterol:**	5mg	**Ratio:**	0.12:1

A hearty and slightly spicy soup packed with prebiotics from sweet potatoes and lentils. Soups are great for cooking in batches.

Benefits: Fiber and Prebiotics
Value: $$
Time: 35 mins
Serves: 6

Ingredients
Thumb-Size (16g) Fresh Ginger
1 Lime
1 Red Delicious Apple (210g)
2 Onions (220g)
3 Garlic Cloves
7 Sweet Potatoes (900g)
1/2 cup (100g) Red Lentils
1 1/4 Cup (20g) Cilantro
10floz (300ml) Whole Milk
1.25qt (1.2L) Vegetable Stock
2 Tsp Medium Curry Powder
3 Tbsp Olive Oil

Method

1. Roughly chop the onions, red apples and ginger, crush the garlic and chop the cilantro stalks.

2. Toast the curry powder in a large saucepan over a medium heat for 2 mins. Add the olive oil, gently stirring as it sizzles. Add the garlic, onions, apple, cilantro stalks and a pinch of salt and pepper. Cook gently for 5 mins, stirring occasionally.

3. Grate the sweet potatoes. Add them into the pan alongside the stock, milk and lentils. Cover and simmer for 20 mins.

4. Blend until creamy. Juice the lime into the soup, check the seasoning and serve. Top with chopped cilantro leaves

Tomato Soup with Pasta

Macronutrients & Omegas per Serving

Kcal:	436	**Carbs:**	62.8g	**Omega 3:**	0.2g
Fat:	13.5g	**Fiber:**	10.4g	**Omega 6:**	1.7g
Protein:	15.7g	**Cholesterol:**	0mg	**Ratio:**	0.12:1

A vegetable packed tomato soup that'll fill you with nutrients as well as prebiotics. The chickpeas, pasta and bread will keep you full until dinner.

Benefits: Fiber & Prebiotics
Value: $
Time: 30 mins
Serves: 4

Ingredients
1 Onion (110g)
2 Celery Sticks (80g)
2 Garlic Cloves
4 Slices (128g) Whole Wheat Bread
2/3 Cup (150g) Orzo Pasta
14oz (400g) Can Chopped Tomatoes
14oz (400g) Can Chickpeas
24floz (700ml) Vegetable Stock
1 Tbsp Tomato Purée
2 Tbsp Basil Pesto
2 Tbsp Olive Oil

Method
1. Heat the olive oil in a large saucepan and chop the onion and celery. Crush the garlic. Fry the onion and celery for 10 mins then add the garlic and cook for 1 more min. Put the pesto and oil aside and stir in all of the other ingredients.

2. Bring to a boil and then reduce the heat and leave to simmer for 6 mins or until the orzo is tender. Season.

3. Mix the pesto with the last tablespoon of oil. Pour the soup into bowls and drizzle the pesto mixture over the soup. Serve with the bread.

Lentil Soup

Macronutrients & Omegas per Serving

Kcal:	313	**Carbs:**	58.8g	**Omega 3:**	0.1g
Fat:	1.9g	**Fiber:**	17.5g	**Omega 6:**	0.6g
Protein:	16.1g	**Cholesterol:**	0mg	**Ratio:**	0.18:1

Another lunch-suitable soup that's extremely easy to prepare and leave to boil for an hour. Leeks and red lentils are the prebiotic powerhouses of this dish, ready to feed your good gut bacteria.

Benefits: Fiber and Prebiotics
Value: $
Time: 1 Hour 10
Serves: 4

Ingredients
2 Large Leeks (270g)
4 Slices (128g) Whole Wheat Bread
6 Carrots (366g)
3/4 Cup (150g) Red Lentils
2qt (2L) Vegetable Stock
2 Tbsp (8g) Parsley

Method
1. Finely chop the carrots and the parsley. Slice the leeks.

2. Add the stock and lentils to a large saucepan and bring to a boil for a few mins.

3. Add the leeks and carrots and season to taste. Bring to a simmer and cover it for 45-60 mins until the lentils are broken down.

4. Scatter with parsley and serve with a slice of buttered whole wheat bread.

Miso Soup

Macronutrients & Omegas per Serving

Kcal:	162	**Carbs:**	21.3g	**Omega 3:**	0.2g
Fat:	4.8g	**Fiber:**	6.4g	**Omega 6:**	2.2g
Protein:	12.9g	**Cholesterol:**	0mg	**Ratio:**	0.07:1

Miso soup is a cheap and quick way to fill your stomach with more healthy probiotics. This soup is the definition of umami.

Benefits: Probiotics
Value: $
Time: 15 mins
Serves: 2

Ingredients
1 Sheet (28g) Dried Seaweed
1/4 Cup (62g) Firm Tofu
1/2 Cup (32g) Swiss Chard
1/2 Cup (45g) Scallion
1qt (950ml) Vegetable Stock
4 Tbsp Miso Paste

Method

1. Chop the swiss chard and scallion. Dice the tofu into cubes.

2. Simmer the vegetable stock in a medium saucepan. Add the dried seaweed and simmer for 5 mins.

3. Place miso into a small bowl and add a little hot water. Whisk until smooth then set aside.

4. Add the swiss chard, scallion and tofu into the saucepan for 5 mins. After cooked, remove from heat and add the resting miso paste. Serve and eat immediately.

Butter Bean & Leek Soup topped with Kale, Toasted Hazelnuts & Bacon

Macronutrients & Omegas per Serving

Kcal:	349	**Carbs:**	34.5g	**Omega 3:**	0.3g
Fat:	19.8g	**Fiber:**	4.3g	**Omega 6:**	2.5g
Protein:	10.8g	**Cholesterol:**	14mg	**Ratio:**	0.1:1

An elaborate soup for those that want a mixture of textures in every bite. It contains a healthy mixture of vegetables, beans, nuts, meat and leafy greens full of prebiotics.

Benefits: Fiber & Prebiotics
Value: $$$
Time: 40 mins
Serves: 4

Ingredients
3 Rashers (84g) Streaky Bacon
5 Leeks (500g)
1/4 Cup (28g) Hazelnuts
2 1/2 Cups (40g) Chopped Kale
2 X 14oz (400g) Can Butter Beans
16floz (500ml) Vegetable Stock
2 Tsp Chopped Thyme
2 Tsp Mustard
1 Tbsp Chopped Parsley
1 Tbsp + 1 Tsp Olive Oil

Method
1. Slice the leeks, chop the hazelnuts and kale whilst removing any tough kale stems.

2. Add 1 tbsp oil into a large saucepan and heat over a low heat. Add the thyme, leeks and seasoning. Cover and cook for 15 mins, the leeks should be soft. If the leeks stick together on the pan, add a splash of water. Add both cans of butter beans, water included, the stock and mustard. Bring to a boil and simmer for 3 mins. Take off the heat and blend to make a soup. Add the parsley, adjust the seasoning if necessary and give it a stir. Keep to one side.

3. Add the bacon to a large, non-stick frying pan and cook until crispy over a medium heat for 3-4 mins. Set the bacon aside to cool but keep the bacon grease in the pan and add the last tsp oil. Add the kale and hazelnuts and cook for 2 mins, stirring until the kale is wilted and crisping at the edges and the hazelnuts are toasted. Cut the cooled bacon into small pieces and add into the kale mixture, stirring thoroughly.

4. When ready to serve, reheat the soup and add some water if too thick. Serve in bowls, placing on top the kale, hazelnut and bacon mixture.

Quinoa Tabbouleh

Macronutrients & Omegas per Serving

Kcal:	315	**Carbs:**	46g	**Omega 3:**	0.1g
Fat:	10.9g	**Fiber:**	7.2g	**Omega 6:**	2.3g
Protein:	10.7g	**Cholesterol:**	0mg	**Ratio:**	0.06:1

A fresh and tangy quinoa-based lunch. Although light, it's sure to refresh and keep you alert for the rest of the afternoon.

Benefits: Fiber and Prebiotics
Value: $$
Time: 40 mins
Serves: 2

Ingredients
1/3 Cucumber (100g)
1/2 Garlic Clove
Juice and Zest 1/2 Lemon
3 Tomatoes (300g)
Drop of Vanilla Extract
Pinch of Himalayan Pink Salt
1/2 Cup (100g) Quinoa
1 1/4 Cup (75g) Chopped Parsley
2 1/2 Cups (50g) Arugula Leaves
1 Tbsp Olive Oil
2 Tbsp Balsamic Vinegar

Method
1. Cut the tomatoes and cucumber into smaller than bite-sized cubes, around 0.5-inch (1cm) and crush the garlic.

2. Cook the quinoa as per its instructions & set aside to cool. Once cooked move onto step 3, if no instructions are present follow the rest of this step. Rinse the quinoa in a fine mesh colander under 30 seconds and drain well to remove the bitterness. Add the quinoa to a saucepan alongside 1 cup water, keep uncovered. Bring to a boil and then simmer for 10 mins or until all the water has been absorbed. Remove from the heat and cover, allowing to steam for 5 mins.

3. Whisk the vinegar, olive oil, lemon juice, vanilla, salt and garlic in a jug until smooth.

4. Mix together with the quinoa and serve on the arugula.

Spring Tabbouleh

Macronutrients & Omegas per Serving

Kcal:	582	**Carbs:**	70.5g	**Omega 3:**	0.2g
Fat:	26.3g	**Fiber:**	16.4g	**Omega 6:**	3.2g
Protein:	18.2g	**Cholesterol:**	0mg	**Ratio:**	0.08:1

A different take on the tabbouleh, raising the fiber content with the addition of both oats and buckwheat. This version includes oven-baking so is perfect for kitchen cleaning multi-tasking. The herbs and lemon add that sharp tabbouleh tang.

Benefits: Fiber and Prebiotics
Value: $$
Time: 45 mins
Serves: 4

Ingredients
1 Cucumber (300g)
2 Lemons, Zested and Juiced
14 Large (250g) Radishes
3/4 Cup (125g) Oats
3/4 Cup (125g) Buckwheat
1 1/2 Cups (240g) Frozen Peas
1/4 Cup (43g) Pomegranate Seeds, To Serve
14oz (400g) Canned Chickpeas
1 Tbsp Garam Masala
4 Tbsp Parsley
4 Tbsp Mint
6 Tbsp Olive Oil

Method
1. Zest and juice the lemons. Chop the radishes, cucumbers, parsley and mint.

2. Preheat the oven to 400°F (200°C)/360°F (180°C) fan/gas 6. Put the chickpeas in a large roast tin, add 4 tbsp oil, garam masala and some seasoning. Thoroughly mix until the chickpeas are coated. Cook for 15 mins, the chickpeas should be starting to crisp. Add the peas, lemon zest, oats and buckwheat, mix thoroughly. Bake for another 10 mins.

3. Transfer to a large mixing bowl and add the herbs, radishes, cucumber, oil and lemon juice. Mix thoroughly. Serve with the pomegranate seeds.

Kale, Bulgur & Hazelnut Tabbouleh

Macronutrients & Omegas per Serving

Kcal:	510	**Carbs:**	75.5g	**Omega 3:**	0.1g
Fat:	15.1g	**Fiber:**	13.9g	**Omega 6:**	2.1g
Protein:	24.5g	**Cholesterol:**	172mg	**Ratio:**	0.06:1

The end of our lunchtime tabbouleh section and this time with bulgur, for its classic taste. The yogurt is added, not only to balance out the dry texture of the bulgur, but to add some probiotics as well.

Benefits: Fiber, Prebiotics and Probiotics
Value: $$
Time: 30 mins
Serves: 2

Ingredients
1/4 Garlic Clove
Juice and Zest 1 Lemon
1 Carrot (60g)
2 Eggs (88g)
3 Scallion (45g)
1/3 Cup (50g) Pomegranate Seeds
3/4 Cup (150g) Bulgur Wheat
3 3/4 Cups (60g) Kale
1 Tsp Chili Flakes
1 Tbsp Chopped Dill
1 Tbsp Chopped Mint
2 Tbsp White Wine Vinegar
2 1/2 Tbsp (20g) Hazelnuts
7 Tbsp Greek Yoghurt

Method
1. If the hazelnuts aren't bought roasted, lay them whole on a cookie sheet and roast at 350°F (175°C) degrees for 15 mins, watching closely as it doesn't take them long to go from brown to burnt. Wait until cooled

then place them in a large clean kitchen towel and rub them until the skins fall off.

2. Chop the hazelnuts, kale, scallions, dill and mint. Julienne (cut into 1/8-inch thick strips) the carrot. Crush the garlic. Cook the bulgur as per its instructions.

3. Bring a pan of water to the boil and add the eggs. Cook for 6 mins, then place in cold water until cool. Peel and cut in half. Put the lemon juice, zest, Greek yogurt, white wine vinegar, dill, mint and garlic into a food processor or blender with 2 tbsp water and some salt. Blend until smooth.

4. Break up the bulgur with a fork and add the hazelnuts, kale, carrots, pomegranate seeds, chili and scallions. Toss with the dressing, then top with the eggs to serve.

Pasta Salad with Tuna

Macronutrients & Omegas per Serving

Kcal:	530	**Carbs:**	74.7g	**Omega 3:**	0.7g
Fat:	14.4g	**Fiber:**	4.4g	**Omega 6:**	1.1g
Protein:	21.9g	**Cholesterol:**	16mg	**Ratio:**	0.63:1

A quick and easy pasta dish that's a surefire way to balance out your Omega levels for the day.

Benefits: Anti-Inflammatory
Value: $
Time: 20 mins
Serves: 4

Ingredients
1 Celery (40g)
15 Peppadew/Cherry/ Peppers (150g)
1/2 Cup (110g) Cherry Tomato
1 Cup (24g) Basil Leaves
3 Cups (350g) Orecchiette Pasta
5 Cups (100g) Arugula Leaves
6oz (170g) Tuna
1 Tbsp Caper
3 Tbsp Olive Oil
5 Tbsp Balsamic Vinegar

Method

1. Chop the peppers, halve the cherry tomatoes and slice the celery.

2. Cook the pasta as per its instructions. Drain and add to a large bowl alongside all other ingredients except the basil. Stir well and serve, topping with basil.

Pomegranate and Broad Bean Salad

Macronutrients & Omegas per Serving

Kcal:	341	**Carbs:**	46.7g	**Omega 3:**	0.1g
Fat:	13.9g	**Fiber:**	9.9g	**Omega 6:**	1.4g
Protein:	10.6g	**Cholesterol:**	0mg	**Ratio:**	0.08:1

A salad packed with herbs that's great for immediate consumption or travel…as long as you store the dressing separately! The pumpkin seeds, fennel and broad beans add some fiber and crunch to the salad.

Benefits: Fiber and Prebiotics
Value: $$
Time: 25 mins
Serves: 6

Ingredients
Small Bunch Mint (10g)
1 Fennel Bulb (230g)
1 Lemon
1 Cup (200g) Bulgur
1 Cup (20g) Arugula
1 1/4 Cups (200g) Pomegranate Seeds
1 1/2 Cups (350g) Broad Beans
1 Tbsp Dijon Mustard
2 Tbsp Chopped Parsley (10g)
2 Tbsp Chopped Dill (10g)
2 Tbsp (16g) Pumpkin Seeds
2 Tbsp Apple Cider Vinegar
5 Tbsp Extra Virgin Olive Oil

Method
1. Finely chop the mint, parsley and dill. Toast the bread. Quarter the fennel bulb, remove the core and thinly slice the quarters.

2. Boil enough water to just about cover the bulgur. Add the bulgur, boiling water and salt to a bowl and cover for 10 mins.

3. If this meal will be eaten at a later date, add the lemon zest, lemon juice, 5 tbs olive oil, 2 tbsp cider vinegar and 1 tbsp mustard to a small transportable container and shake vigorously. Otherwise add these ingredients to a bowl and stir thoroughly.

4. Uncover the bulgur. If there is any water left, drain it. Add the fennel, herbs, pomegranate seeds, broad beans and pumpkin seeds and mix thoroughly. Top with the Arugula.

5. When ready to serve, drizzle the dressing and mix everything thoroughly.

Pesto Chicken Salad

Macronutrients & Omegas per Serving

Kcal:	456	**Carbs:**	15.6g	**Omega 3:**	1g
Fat:	24g	**Fiber:**	6.7g	**Omega 6:**	4.9g
Protein:	49g	**Cholesterol:**	158mg	**Ratio:**	0.2:1

The star of the show is the homemade avocado pesto. It's delicious and will teach you how to make pesto, that's both cheaper and fresher than store bought, with the added benefit of balancing out your Omegas.

Benefits: Fiber, Prebiotics & Anti-Inflammatory
Value: $$$
Time: 30 mins
Serves: 4

Ingredients
1 Red Onion (148g)
1 1/2 (250g) Broccoli
2 Raw Beets (165g)
3 Skinless Chicken Breasts (543g)
1 Cup (100g) Watercress
1 Tsp Flax Seeds
1 Tbsp + 2 Tsp Olive Oil

Avocado Pesto (or use store bought):
1/2 Garlic Clove
Juice and Zest 1/2 Lemon
1 Avocado (150g), Stoned & Peeled
1/4 Cup (25g) Walnuts
1 1/3 Cup (32g) Basil

Method
1. Grate the raw beets, crush the garlic, crumble the walnuts and thinly slice the red onion.

2. Boil the broccoli in a large saucepan for 2 mins. Drain then finish it off in a gridle or frying pan for 2-3 mins alongside 1/2 tsp olive oil. Set aside to cool.

3. Brush the chicken with 1 1/2 tsp of olive oil and either gridle or fry until cooked through, roughly 3-4 mins each side. Put to one side then slice once cooled.

4. For the avocado pesto, pick the leaves from the basil and add the rest into a food processor. Add the avocado, garlic, walnuts, 1 tbsp oil, 1 tbsp lemon juice, 2 tbsp cold water and some seasoning. Blend until it turns to a smooth paste.

5. Put the sliced red onion on a plate and pour over the rest of the lemon juice, leaving to stand for a few mins.

6. In a large mixing bowl, toss the watercress, broccoli, onion and lemon juice from the bottom of the plate.

7. Serve the salad mix from the mixing bowl. Top with beetroot, chicken, basil leaves, lemon zest and flax seeds. Put the pesto in a small bowl that can be shared.

Beetroot & Chickpea Pita

Macronutrients & Omegas per Serving

Kcal:	275	**Carbs:**	52.5g	**Omega 3:**	0g
Fat:	3.1g	**Fiber:**	9.6g	**Omega 6:**	0.6g
Protein:	11.7g	**Cholesterol:**	3mg	**Ratio:**	0.05:1

This quick pita recipe is ideally made and eaten immediately. However, if planning to store in a lunchbox and eat later in the day, make sure to store the filling separately from the pita to prevent it from getting soggy.

Benefits: Fiber
Value: $
Time: 30 mins/10 min with pre-boiled beet
Serves: 2

Ingredients
1 Small Carrot (40g)
1 Beet (80g)
2 Large (130g) Whole Wheat Pita
4oz (120g) Canned Chickpeas
1 Tsp Harissa
2 Tbsp Greek Yogurt

Method

1. Boil the beet for 30-60 mins depending on the size. It should be tender enough for a fork to go through but not soft and mushy.

2. Grate the beet and carrot into a bowl. Add the chickpeas, harissa and 1 tbsp Greek yogurt. Mix together with the backside of a fork. Alternatively add this mixture to a blender and blend until a hummus like texture.

3. Cut an opening in the middle of the pitas and add the mixture. Garnish with 1 tbsp Greek yogurt.

Veggie Club Sandwich

Macronutrients & Omegas per Serving

Kcal:	488	**Carbs:**	61.1g	**Omega 3:**	0.2g
Fat:	20.9g	**Fiber:**	12.4g	**Omega 6:**	3g
Protein:	17.9g	**Cholesterol:**	0mg	**Ratio:**	0.08:1

Another – perfect for the lunchbox – treat, as long as the wet hummus mixture is kept away from the bread until serving of course!

Benefits: Fiber
Value: $
Time: 10 mins
Serves: 1

Ingredients
Small Squeeze Lemon Juice
1 Carrot (60g)
2 Tomatoes (246g)
3 Slices (96g) Whole Wheat Bread
1 Cup (35g) Watercress
1 Tbsp Olive Oil
2 Tbsp Hummus

Method
1. Grate the carrot and cut the tomatoes into thick slices. Toast the bread.

2. Mix the carrot, watercress, lemon juice and olive oil together in a small bowl.

3. After the bread is toasted, spread the hummus over each slice of toast.

4. Top 1 slice (hummus side up) with half the watercress mixture & tomatoes, then add the next slice and repeat one more time. Make sure the final slice is hummus side down, press down and slice into quarters.

Spicy Chicken Avocado Wraps

Macronutrients & Omegas per Serving

Kcal:	563	**Carbs:**	44.2g	**Omega 3:**	0.2g
Fat:	27.6g	**Fiber:**	14.4g	**Omega 6:**	3.3g
Protein:	38.4g	**Cholesterol:**	105mg	**Ratio:**	0.07:1

Leftover chicken in the fridge? Time to pair it with some avocado and bell pepper, wrapped in a whole wheat tortilla for a high protein and fiber lunch.

Benefits: Fiber and Prebiotics
Value: $$$
Time: 15 mins
Serves: 2

Ingredients
1/2 Juice Lime
1 Chicken Breast (180g), Thinly Sliced at An Angle
1 Garlic Clove
1 Avocado (175g), Stoned & Peeled
1 Red Bell Pepper (120g)
2 Large Whole Wheat Wraps (140g)
1/2 Tsp Mild Chili Powder
1 Tsp Olive Oil
1 Tbsp Cilantro

Method

1. Chop the garlic and cilantro. Thinly slice the bell pepper and chicken.

2. Add the chicken breast to a bowl alongside the chili powder, garlic and lime juice. Stir thoroughly so the chicken is coated.

3. Add the oil to a non-stick frying pan and fry the chicken for a few mins until warmed through.

4. Simultaneously warm the wraps on a gas stove top or in the microwave as per its instructions.

5. Add the peppers to the frying pan. Squash half an avocado to each wrap and then evenly split the contents of the frying pan into each wrap. Top with cilantro, roll the wraps and serve.

Crunchy Chickpea & Avocado Wraps

Macronutrients & Omegas per Serving

Kcal:	596	**Carbs:**	66.5g	**Omega 3:**	0.2g
Fat:	28.7g	**Fiber:**	22.7g	**Omega 6:**	2.8g
Protein:	19g	**Cholesterol:**	5mg	**Ratio:**	0.08:1

For the days where you can't seem to get your recommended fiber, fear not. This recipe catapults you towards your 20-38g recommended fiber intake per day. If the combination of chickpeas and whole wheat tortillas is a little dry for your palette, liberally add more Greek yogurt or avocado.

Benefits: Fiber, Prebiotics and Probiotics
Value: $$
Time: 45 mins
Serves: 4

Ingredients
Small Pack Cilantro (10g)
1 Lime
2 Large Avocados (400g), Stoned & Peeled
8 Whole Wheat Tortillas (330g)
10 Roasted Red Bell Peppers from a Jar
1/2 Cup (150g) Greek Yogurt
8 Cups Kale (130g)
14oz (400g) Can Chickpeas
2 Tsp Olive Oil
2 Tsp Ground Cumin
2 Tsp Smoked Paprika
1 Tsp Chili Powder

Method

1. Stone, peel and chop the avocados. Juice the lime. Chop the cilantro and roasted red peppers and the shred the lettuce.

2. Heat oven to 425°F (220°C)/400°F (200°C) fan/gas 7. Drain the chickpeas and pour them in a large bowl. Add the olive oil, cumin, paprika and chili. Stir the chickpeas well to coat, then spread them onto a large baking tray and roast for 20-25 mins or until starting to crisp – give the tray a shake halfway through cooking to ensure they roast evenly. Remove from the oven and season to taste.

3. Toss the chopped avocados with the lime juice and chopped cilantro, then set aside until serving.

4. Warm the tortillas following pack instructions, then pile in the avocado, kale, yogurt, peppers and toasted chickpeas at the table. Add more yogurt if needed to balance out the texture of the chickpeas and tortilla.

Spanish Sweet Potato Tortilla (Omelet)

Macronutrients & Omegas per Serving

Kcal:	416	**Carbs:**	33.7g	**Omega 3:**	0.3g
Fat:	26g	**Fiber:**	5.9g	**Omega 6:**	3g
Protein:	13.4g	**Cholesterol:**	273mg	**Ratio:**	0.09:1

A Spanish style tortilla filled with sweet potato and spinach that will feed you and a partner for 2-3 lunches. Filled with protein from the eggs and fiber from the sweet potatoes.

Benefits: Fiber and Prebiotics
Value: $$
Time: 1 Hour 10
Serves: 6

Ingredients
2 Garlic Cloves, Thinly Sliced
2 Large Onions (275g), Thinly Sliced
4 Medium Sweet Potatoes, Thinly Sliced (1lb 12oz/800g)
8 Large Eggs (440g)
10 Cups (300g) Baby Spinach Leaves
8 Tbsp Olive Oil

Method
1. Heat 3 tbsp oil to a lidded large non-stick pan over a low-medium heat. Add the onions and cover for 15 mins, they should be soft but remain their color.

2. Boil some water. Add the spinach into a large colander and gently pour the boiling water all over it. Allow to cool, drain well and squeeze a little more water out of the spinach without crunching it too much. Separate any clumps gently.

3. Add 3 more tbsp oil, garlic and potatoes, season generously and mix thoroughly. Cover and cook for an additional 15 mins until the potatoes are very soft, stirring occasionally.

4. In a large bowl, whisk the eggs and add the cooked potato mixture, stirring thoroughly. Add the spinach and fold gently, keeping the soft potato intact.

5. Add 2 tbsp oil to the empty pan and pour back in the sweet potato egg mixture. Cover and cook the mixture over a low-medium heat for 20 mins. The base and sides should turn golden and the center should almost set. With a spatula, gently separate the sides from the pan to stop if from sticking.

6. Get a large plate, cover the tortilla and flip it. Return the tortilla back to the pan and cook for an additional 5 mins uncovered until the egg is fully set and its golden everywhere. If it breaks a little during the flip, it will set again in the final 5 mins of cooking. Use the spatula to separate the sides from the pan again.

7. Rest for 5 mins and then slide it onto a plate or board. Cut into wedges and serve.

Chicken, Spinach & Hummus Bowl

Macronutrients & Omegas per Serving

Kcal:	580	**Carbs:**	50.6g	**Omega 3:**	0.2g
Fat:	25g	**Fiber:**	15.9g	**Omega 6:**	2.8g
Protein:	45.5g	**Cholesterol:**	105mg	**Ratio:**	0.08:1

Another great dish for leftovers, quinoa and brown rice in particular. If you're feeling particularly artistic, keep all ingredients in each bowl separate and serve, allowing your guest the satisfaction of mixing everything together themselves.

Benefits: Fiber and Prebiotics
Value: $$
Time: 10 mins
Serves: 2

Ingredients
1/2 Red Onion (75g)
1 Small Lemon, Zested and Juiced
1 Small Avocado (100g), Stoned & Peeled
1 Cooked Chicken Breast (180g)
1/4 Cup (33g) Quinoa
1/3 Cup (33g) Brown Rice
1/2 Cup (100g) Pomegranate Seeds
1 1/4 Cups (200g) Hummus
6oz (170g) Baby Spinach
2 Tbsp Toasted Almonds

Method

1. Cook the quinoa and brown rice as per its instructions.

2. Chop the spinach, slice the avocado, finely slice the red onion and slice the chicken breast at an angle.

3. In a small bowl, add 2 tbsp hummus, half the lemon juice, all of the lemon zest and 1 tsp water. Mix thoroughly. The hummus should be of a consistency that allows it to be drizzled, but not too watery. Add additional water if need be.

4. In two bowls, evenly split the brown rice and quinoa. Add the hummus dressing and mix thoroughly. Top with spinach.

5. Squeeze the rest of the lemon juice over the avocado and add them to the bowl. Finally, add the chicken, pomegranate seeds, onion, almonds and remaining hummus. Mix both bowls thoroughly and serve.

Black-Eyed Pea Mole with Salsa

Macronutrients & Omegas per Serving

Kcal:	279	**Carbs:**	46.1g	**Omega 3:**	0.1g
Fat:	6.3g	**Fiber:**	13.9g	**Omega 6:**	0.9g
Protein:	13.4g	**Cholesterol:**	0mg	**Ratio:**	0.16:1

Home-made salsa and mole are an effortless way to get some fresh vegetables and spices into your system. Onions, tomatoes and black-eyed peas are the key to adding fiber and prebiotics.

Benefits: Fiber and Prebiotics
Value: $
Time: 25 mins
Serves: 2

Ingredients
1/2 Lime, Zest and Juice
1 Garlic Clove
2 Red Onion (300g)
2 Large Tomatoes (300g)
9oz (250g) Black-Eyed Peas
1/2 Tsp Ground Cinnamon
1 Tsp Vegetable Bouillon Powder
1 Tsp Ground Cilantro
1 Tsp Mild Chili Powder
2 Tsp Cocoa
2 Tsp Olive Oil
1 Tbsp Tomato Purée
2 Tbsp Fresh Cilantro

Method
1. Finely chop one red onion, halve and slice the other. Finely grate the garlic and chop both tomatoes.

2. Add the finely chopped red onion, tomatoes, 2 tbsp cilantro, lime zest and juice into a bowl and stir thoroughly.

3. In a non-stick pan heat 2 tsp olive oil. On a medium-high heat fry the onion and garlic until softened, stirring frequently. Add the rest of the cilantro, chili powder and ground cinnamon and stir thoroughly.

4. Add the can of black-eyed peas as well as their water, the cocoa, vegetable bouillon and tomato puree. Make sure the sauce becomes thick by stirring frequently.

5. Serve the mole into shallow bowls and top with your salsa.

Dinner

Chicken & Sweet Potato Curry

Macronutrients & Omegas per Serving

Kcal:	378	**Carbs:**	34.3g	**Omega 3:**	0.3g
Fat:	16.2g	**Fiber:**	7g	**Omega 6:**	4.3g
Protein:	26.3g	**Cholesterol:**	185mg	**Ratio:**	0.06:1

The curry paste can be swapped for any other kind, making this sweet potato curry customizable to your heat tolerance. A quick and easy mid-week meal.

Benefits: Fiber and Prebiotics
Value: $$
Time: 30 mins
Serves: 4

Ingredients

1 Large Red Onion (185g)
2 Large Tomatoes (300g)
4 Sweet Potatoes (500g)
4 Skinless Chicken Thigh Fillets (480g)
4 Cups (120g) Spinach
1 Tbsp Olive Oil
2 Tbsp Rogan Josh Curry Paste

Method

1. Cut the sweet potato into 1-inch (2cm) cubes and the chicken and tomatoes into bite-sized pieces. Chop the tomatoes and cut the red onion into wedges.

2. Boil the sweet potatoes until tender for roughly 12 mins and then drain and set aside.

3. Heat 1 tbsp oil in a large frying pan and cook the chicken and onion together for 5 mins, until the chicken is cooked through. Add the curry paste, stir thoroughly and cook for 1 more min, add the tomatoes and cook for 1 last min.

4. Add 3fl oz of boiling water to the frying pan and mix. Simmer for 5 mins then add the spinach and sweet potatoes and cook for an additional 2 mins. Serve either by itself or with brown rice.

Smoky Tomato & Bacon Spaghetti

Macronutrients & Omegas per Serving

Kcal:	558	**Carbs:**	80.4g	**Omega 3:**	0.1g
Fat:	17.6g	**Fiber:**	18.5g	**Omega 6:**	2.3g
Protein:	18.3g	**Cholesterol:**	20mg	**Ratio:**	0.05:1

Swapping regular spaghetti for a whole wheat version doubles the amount of fiber, making this tasty meal suitable for diverticular disease patients. This recipe contains a sneaky secret for thickening up sauces, add a ladle of pasta water!

Benefits: Fiber and Prebiotics
Value: $
Time: 25 mins
Serves: 4

Ingredients
1 Onion (110g)
2 Garlic Cloves
4 Slices (120g) Smoked Streaky Bacon
14oz (400g) Whole Wheat Spaghetti
2 X 14oz (400g) Cans Chopped Tomatoes
1 Tbsp Sweet Smoked Paprika
1 Tbsp Olive Oil

Method
1. Boil the spaghetti as per packet instructions. Slice the bacon into thin slices vertically and then into thirds horizontally. Finely chop the onion and garlic.

2. Heat 1 tbsp oil in a large non-stick pan and cook the bacon until it starts to crisp for 3-4 mins on a medium heat. Add the onion and cook for 4 mins then add the garlic and smoked paprika for 1 more min.

3. Pour in the chopped tomatoes and one ladle of pasta water, simmering for 5 mins until thick. Stir occasionally. Mix in the drained pasta and serve with grated cheese if you'd like.

Greek-Style Roast Fish

Macronutrients & Omegas per Serving

Kcal:	492	**Carbs:**	63g	**Omega 3:**	0.6g
Fat:	15.7g	**Fiber:**	7.1g	**Omega 6:**	1.6g
Protein:	27.6g	**Cholesterol:**	71mg	**Ratio:**	0.37:1

Although there are many great potatoes for roasting such as Yukon Gold or Maris Pipers, Russet potatoes come in at the higher spectrum of the fiber per potato ratio. Pollock or any other oily fish is a great addition to balance out your daily Omegas.

Benefits: Fiber, Prebiotics and Anti-Inflammatory
Value: $$
Time: 1 Hour 10
Serves: 2
Ingredients
1/2 Lemon
Small Handful Parsley
2 Large Tomatoes (300g)
2 Fresh Pollock Fillets (200g)
2 Onions (220g)
3 Garlic Cloves, Roughly Chopped
3 Small Russet (or Maris Piper) Potatoes (500g)
1/2 Tsp Dried Oregano
2 Tbsp Olive Oil

Method

1. Preheat oven to 400°F (200°C)/350°F (180 °C) fan/gas 6. Scrub the potato then cut it into quarter wedges before parboiling them for 10 mins in salty water. Cut the lemon and tomatoes into wedges, halve and slice the onions then chop the garlic and parsley.

2. Add the parboiled potatoes, oregano and olive oil into a roasting tin, season, then mix together with your hands to coat everything in the oil.

Roast for 15 mins then turn everything over and add the onion and garlic, baking for 15 mins more.

3. Add the lemon and tomatoes and roast for 10 mins, then top with the fish fillets and cook for 10-12 mins until the fish is soft. Serve with parsley scattered over.

Chinese Curry Chicken

Macronutrients & Omegas per Serving

Kcal:	494	**Carbs:**	46.1g	**Omega 3:**	0.1g
Fat:	16.4g	**Fiber:**	6.9g	**Omega 6:**	1.6g
Protein:	42.1g	**Cholesterol:**	90mg	**Ratio:**	0.08:1

This recipe takes the "velveting" Chinese secret and makes it suitable for home-cooking. Velveting is the technique of coating chicken and quickly frying it to seal in its juices. The Chinese restaurant approach requires enough oil to fully submerge the chicken, so this recipe makes it home-cook friendly by switching that final step for blanching, i.e. parboiling the chicken.

Benefits: Fiber and Prebiotics
Value: $$
Time: 1 Hour
Serves: 4

Ingredients
Pinch Sugar
1 Onion (110g)
1 Garlic Clove
2 Egg Whites (50g)
4 Skinless Chicken Breasts (600g)
2 Cups (320g) Frozen Peas
3 Cups (300g) Brown Rice
13.5floz (400ml) Chicken Stock
1/2 Tsp Ground Ginger
1 Tsp Turmeric
1 Tsp Soy Sauce
2 Tsp Salt
2 Tsp Curry Powder
2 Tbsp Cornstarch
3 Tbsp Olive Oil

Method

1. Cook the brown rice as per its instructions. Whisk the egg whites, cornstarch and salt in a bowl until smooth. Cut the chicken breasts into chunks and coat them in the marinade, marinating in the fridge for 30 mins. Bring a pot of water to boil, add 1 tbsp olive oil and turn to a medium heat. Remove excess coating and add directly to boiling water for 1 min, just enough to keep the marinade coating intact, and then drain and set aside. The chicken should be opaque. It is ok if there are small clumps of egg white or cornstarch.

2. Dice the onion and crush the garlic. Fry the onion in a wok on low to medium heat for 5 mins until they soften, then add the garlic and cook for 1 min. Stir in the spices and sugar and cook for another minute, add the stock and soy sauce, bring to a simmer and cook for 20 minutes. Tip everything into a blender and blend until smooth.

3. Fry the chicken in the remaining oil until it is browned all over. Tip the sauce back into the pan and bring everything to a simmer, stir in the peas and cook for 5 minutes. Add a little water if you need to thin the sauce. Serve with brown rice.

Pea, Paneer & Cauliflower Curry

Macronutrients & Omegas per Serving

Kcal:	510	**Carbs:**	53.3g	**Omega 3:**	0.1g
Fat:	23g	**Fiber:**	13.7g	**Omega 6:**	1.4g
Protein:	24.1g	**Cholesterol:**	1mg	**Ratio:**	0.05:1

The curry paste can be exchanged for one to your liking, giving this dish a big reusability factor. The cauliflower, peas and naan give this recipe the kick of fiber it needs.

Benefits: Fiber and Prebiotics
Value: $
Time: 1 Hour
Serves: 4

Ingredients
Small Pack (10g) Cilantro
1 Head (600g) of Cauliflower
2 Onions (220g)
2 Whole Wheat Naan (210g)
3 Garlic Cloves
2 Cups (250g) Paneer Cheese
7oz (200g) Frozen Peas
17.5oz (500g) Passata/Strained Tomatoes
2 Tbsp Olive Oil
2 Heaped Tbsp Tikka Masala Paste
Raita or Chutney, To Serve

Method

1. Chop the cauliflower into small pieces, cut the paneer cheese into medium-large cubes, thickly slice the onions, crush the garlic and chop the cilantro.

2. Heat 1 tbsp of oil in a large non-stick frying pan and fry the paneer cheese gently until crisp. Remove with a slotted spoon and set aside.

Add the remaining oil and the cauliflower to the pan and cook until browned, roughly 10 mins for small pieces. Add the onions, and a little more oil if needed, and cook for a further 5 mins until softened. Stir in the garlic and curry paste, then pour in the passata, 8.5floz (250ml) water and add some season. Bring to a simmer, then cover and cook for 18-20 mins or until the cauliflower is just tender. If the cauliflower wasn't cut small enough it may take additional time.

3. Add the frozen peas and crispy paneer to the pan and cook for a further 5 mins. Stir through most of the cilantro and garnish with the rest. Serve with naan bread and some minty raita or your favorite chutney.

Asparagus, Pea & Broad Bean Shakshuka

Macronutrients & Omegas per Serving

Kcal:	333	**Carbs:**	35.5g	**Omega 3:**	0.1g
Fat:	15.8g	**Fiber:**	12.2g	**Omega 6:**	1.8g
Protein:	21.8g	**Cholesterol:**	207mg	**Ratio:**	0.08:1

Shakshuka is a Middle Eastern and North African dish that combines tomatoes with spices and then poaches the eggs in this flavorful mixture. The whole wheat flatbread brings a large amount of fiber and the Greek yogurt adds the probiotics.

Benefits: Fiber, Prebiotics and Probiotics
Value: $$
Time: 50 mins
Serves: 4

Ingredients
2 Scallions (30g)
4 Ripe Tomatoes (500g)
4 Large Eggs (220g)
4 Whole Wheat Flatbreads, To Serve
8 Asparagus Spears (125g)
1/3 Cup (50g) Peas
1/4 Cup (60g) Broad Beans
7oz (200g) Broccoli
2 Tbsp Olive Oil
2 Tbsp Chopped Parsley
4 Tbsp Greek Yogurt, To Serve
Large Pinch Cayenne Pepper, Plus Extra to Serve

Method
1. Remove the woody end of the asparagus then finely slice the spears, leaving 1-inch (2cm) intact at the top. Finely slice the broccoli, leaving the heads and 1-inch (2cm) of stalk intact. Finely slice the scallions then chop the tomatoes.

2. Heat the oil in a frying pan. Add the scallions, asparagus and broccoli and fry gently until they soften a little, then add the cumin seeds, cayenne, tomatoes (with their juices), parsley and plenty of seasoning, and stir. Cover with a lid and cook for 5 mins to make a base sauce, then add the broccoli heads, cover and cook for an additional 2 mins. Add the asparagus spears, peas and broad beans, cover again and cook for 2 more mins.

3. Make 4 dips in the mixture. Break an egg into each dip, season well, cover with a lid and cook until the egg whites are just set. Serve with a spoonful of yogurt and some flatbreads, and sprinkle over another pinch of cayenne, if you like.

Veggie Curry

Macronutrients & Omegas per Serving

Kcal:	457	**Carbs:**	77.4g	**Omega 3:**	0.2g
Fat:	10.5g	**Fiber:**	15.7g	**Omega 6:**	1.4g
Protein:	17.9g	**Cholesterol:**	0mg	**Ratio:**	0.15:1

Adding a curry spin to the chili con carne classic. This recipe is very high in fiber and prebiotics thanks to the veg, beans and brown rice.

Benefits: Fiber and Prebiotics
Value: $
Time: 35 mins
Serves: 2

Ingredients
(Optional) 1/2 Red Chili Pepper (23g)
Thumb-Sized Piece of Ginger (16g)
1 Onion (110g)
2 Garlic Cloves
2/3 Cup (10g) Cilantro, including Stalks and Leaves
1 1/2 Cup (150g) Brown Rice
14oz (400g) Can Chopped Tomatoes
14oz (400g) Can Kidney Beans
1 Tsp Ground Cumin
1 Tsp Ground Paprika
2 Tsp Curry Paste
1 Tbsp Olive Oil

Method

1. Cook the brown rice as per its instructions.

2. Peel the ginger and finely chop it alongside the onion, garlic and chili. Finely chop the cilantro stalks and shred its leaves.

3. Heat the oil in a large frying pan over a low-medium heat. Add the onion and a pinch of salt and cook slowly, stirring occasionally, until softened and just starting to color. Add the garlic, ginger and cilantro stalks and cook for a further 2 mins, until fragrant.

4. Add the spices to the pan and cook for another 1 min. Tip in the chopped tomatoes, kidney beans alongside their water and chili then bring to the boil.

5. Turn down the heat and simmer for 15 mins until the curry is nice and thick. Season to taste, then serve with the cooked brown rice and cilantro leaves.

Curried Cod

Macronutrients & Omegas per Serving

Kcal:	477	**Carbs:**	52.7g	**Omega 3:**	1.1g
Fat:	14.3g	**Fiber:**	11.4g	**Omega 6:**	1.6g
Protein:	34.7g	**Cholesterol:**	71mg	**Ratio:**	0.72:1

Trout has a very fishy taste which may not appeal to everyone's palate but fear not, a well-spiced curry can mask the flavor whilst maintaining the incredible amount of Omega 3s.

Benefits: Fiber, Prebiotics and Anti-Inflammatory
Value: $$
Time: 35 mins
Serves: 4
Ingredients
Handful Cilantro
Thumb-Sized Piece Ginger (16g)
1/2 Red Chili Pepper (23g)
1 Onion (110g)
1 Lemon
4 Garlic Cloves
6 Skinless Trout Fillets (480g)
3 Cups (300g) Brown Rice
14oz (400g) Can Chickpeas
2 X 14oz (400g) Cans Chopped Tomatoes
1 Tbsp Olive Oil
2 Tbsp Medium Curry Powder

Method

1. Cook the brown rice as per its instructions.

2. Peel and finely grate the ginger, chop the onions and cilantro, crush the garlic, zest the lemon and then cut into wedges.

3. Heat the oil in a large, lidded frying pan. Cook the onion over a high heat for a few mins, then stir in the curry powder, ginger and garlic.

Cook for another 1-2 mins until fragrant, then stir in the tomatoes, chickpeas and some seasoning.

4. Cook for 8-10 mins until thickened slightly, then top with the cod. Cover and cook for another 5-10 mins until the fish is cooked through. Scatter over the lemon zest and cilantro, then serve with the lemon wedges to squeeze over.

Roast Sea Bass with a Lemony Sweet Potato Salad

Macronutrients & Omegas per Serving

Kcal:	400	**Carbs:**	52.7g	**Omega 3:**	1.1g
Fat:	8g	**Fiber:**	9.9g	**Omega 6:**	0.5g
Protein:	30.3g	**Cholesterol:**	54mg	**Ratio:**	1.92:1

Another fish dish to keep your gut glad. Packed with Omega 3s from the sea bass as well as fiber and prebiotics from the sweet potatoes. Using the whole lemon, zest and juice, gives the dish a citrus twist.

Benefits: Fiber, Prebiotics and Anti-Inflammatory
Value: $$
Time: 1 hour 30 mins
Serves: 2

Ingredients
1 Lemon
1 Garlic Clove
2 Sea Bass Fillets (260g)
2 Large Sweet Potatoes (350g)
2 Red Onions (300g)
1/4 Cup (45g) Pomegranate Seeds
4.5oz (125g) Baby Spinach
1 Tsp Fennel Seeds
2 Tsp Extra Virgin Olive Oil
3 Tbsp Chopped Parsley

Method
1. Heat oven to 350°F (180°C)/325°F (160°C) fan/gas 4. Cut the red onions into wedges. Scrub the sweet potatoes and cut into cubes. Put in a roasting tin with the onions, fennel, and 6 whole garlic cloves, then toss with the oil. Put the potatoes in the oven and roast for 25mins, turning everything over halfway through.

2. Zest the whole lemon and then slice it in half. Cut one half into rounds. Put the fish fillets on top of the roasted potatoes and place the lemon rounds on the fish. Roast for 5 mins.

3. Finely chop the garlic. Squeeze the other half of the lemon into a bowl and mix it with the lemon zest, parsley, garlic, oil and some black pepper.

4. Remove the potatoes and fish from the oven. Temporarily take the fish off, stir in the spinach and add the fillets back on top. Roast for 2 more mins.

5. Remove the fish and potatoes from the oven. Place one sea bass fillet on each plate. Add the lemon mixture and pomegranate seeds to the potatoes, spinach and onions and toss thoroughly. Serve the salad, placing the fillets to one side or on top.

Grilled Tuna Steaks with Quinoa Salad & Mint Chutney

Macronutrients & Omegas per Serving

Kcal:	609	**Carbs:**	42.6g	**Omega 3:**	3g
Fat:	17.5g	**Fiber:**	6.4g	**Omega 6:**	1.4g
Protein:	67.8g	**Cholesterol:**	97mg	**Ratio:**	2.22:1

A minty yogurt marinade transforms delicious tuna steaks into a Probiotic & Anti-Inflammatory contender not to be messed with! Accompanied by some vegetables and quinoa for the much-needed fiber, this recipe includes everything you need to cover in a diverticular diet.

Benefits: Fiber, Prebiotics, Probiotics and Anti-Inflammatory
Value: $$$
Time: 30 mins
Serves: 2

Ingredients
1/4 Cucumber (75g)
Good Squeeze of Lemon Juice
Pinch of Cumin Seeds
1 Garlic Clove
1 Small Red Onion (100g)
4 Tomatoes (500g)
1/3 Cup (60g) Quinoa
1/2 Cup (150g) Greek Yogurt
4 X 4oz (115g) Thin Tuna Steaks
1/4 Tsp Turmeric
3 Tbsp Chopped Mint
3 Tbsp Chopped Cilantro

Method
1. Put 2 tbsp of the mint and cilantro in a bowl. Add the yogurt and garlic, and blitz with a hand blender until smooth. Stir 2 tbsp of the

herby yogurt with the turmeric and cumin, then add the fish and turn in the mixture to completely coat. Marinate in a closed bag for at least 15 mins, preferably an hour.

2. Boil the quinoa as per its instructions. Drain well.

3. Chop the mint, cilantro, and tomatoes. Finely chop the red onion and finely dice the cucumber.

4. Preheat the oven broiler/grill to high. If placing the fish on a grill grate, lightly oil the grate first. Arrange the fish in a shallow heatproof dish and grill for 5-7 mins per side, depending on thickness, until it flakes.

5. Toss the quinoa with the cucumber, onion, tomatoes, lemon juice and remaining herbs. Spoon onto a plate, add the fish and spoon round the mint chutney, or add it at the table.

Garlic Turkey Meatballs with Vegetable Sauce

Macronutrients & Omegas per Serving

Kcal:	392	**Carbs:**	41.5g	**Omega 3:**	0.1g
Fat:	10.5g	**Fiber:**	8g	**Omega 6:**	1.2g
Protein:	34.4g	**Cholesterol:**	66mg	**Ratio:**	0.06:1

Turkey is a leaner counterpart to its chicken rival but is ideal for poultry meatballs! A wholesome vegetable dish at its heart with plenty of flavor.

Benefits: Fiber and Prebiotics
Value: $$
Time: 1 Hour
Serves: 4

Ingredients
1 Onion (110g)
1 Fennel Bulb (234g)
1 Broccoli (150g)
2 Carrots (120g)
2 Celery Sticks (80g)
3 Garlic Cloves
14oz (400g) Lean Ground Turkey Breast
17.5oz (500g) Passata/Strained Tomatoes
1.5lb (700g) New/Baby Potatoes
17floz (500ml) Chicken Stock
1 Tsp Fennel Seed
2 Tbsp Chopped Parsley
2 Tbsp Olive Oil
4 Tbsp (22g) Oats

Method

1. Finely chop the onion and 2 garlic cloves then finely dice the carrots and celery. Halve the fennel bulb and thinly slice, keeping the fronds (feathery leaves at the top). Crush the tsp fennel seeds and 1 garlic.

Chop the broccoli into bite-sized pieces and remove the hard part of the stalk.

2. Heat 1 tbsp oil in a large non-stick frying pan with a lid, then tip in the onion, carrots, celery, garlic and fennel, and stir well. Cover the pan and cook over a medium heat for 8 mins, stirring every now and then. Pour in the passata/strained tomatoes and stock, cover and leave to simmer for 20 mins.

3. Place the new/baby potatoes in a pan of boiling water and gently simmer for 15-20 mins until tender.

4. Tip the mince into a large bowl. Add the oats, fennel seeds and leaves, the garlic and plenty of black pepper, and mix in with your hands. Shape into 25 meatballs about the size of a walnut. Heat 1 tbsp olive oil in a non-stick pan and gently cook the meatballs until they take on a little color. Give the sauce a stir, then add the meatballs and parsley. Cover and cook for 3 mins, then add the broccoli and cook for another 7 mins until the meatballs are cooked through and the veg in the sauce is tender.

5. Serve together with the drained baby potatoes, adding a little butter if you desire.

Layered Eggplant & Lentil Bake

Macronutrients & Omegas per Serving

Kcal:	456	**Carbs:**	57.5g	**Omega 3:**	0.3g
Fat:	18.8g	**Fiber:**	14.3g	**Omega 6:**	1.5g
Protein:	21g	**Cholesterol:**	25mg	**Ratio:**	0.18:1

A fibrous vegetarian style meal that contains a large amount of protein from lentils. The mozzarella can be exchanged for a nut or soy-based cheese to make the recipe vegan friendly.

Benefits: Fiber & Prebiotics
Value: $
Time: 1 hour
Serves: 4

Ingredients
Small Pack (5g) Basil Leaves
2 Eggplant (800g)
2 Onions (220g)
3 Garlic Cloves
3/4 Cup (145g) Green Lentils
2 Cups Butternut Squash Cubes (300g)
4.5oz (125g) Ball of Mozzarella
14oz (400g) Can Chopped Tomatoes
3 Tbsp Olive Oil

Method
1. Cut eggplant into 1/4-inch (0.5 cm) slices lengthways. Finely chop the onions and garlic and dice the butternut squash.

2. Heat oven to 425°F (220°C)/400°F (200°C) fan/gas 7. Brush both sides of the eggplant with 2 tbsp olive oil and lay alongside the squash on baking sheets. Season and bake for 15-20 mins until tender, turning once.

3. Cook the lentils following its instructions.

4. Heat the remaining oil in a large frying pan. Tip in the onions and garlic and cook until soft. Add the tomatoes, plus ½ can of water. Simmer for 10-15 mins until the sauce has thickened. Stir in the lentils, basil and seasoning.

5. Spoon a layer of lentils into a small baking dish. Top with eggplant slices, then lentils and repeat, finishing with a layer of eggplant. Scatter with torn mozzarella pieces and bake for a further 15 mins until the cheese is golden and bubbling.

Tomato, Sweet Potato & Zucchini Stew

Macronutrients & Omegas per Serving

Kcal:	299	**Carbs:**	55.1g	**Omega 3:**	0.2g
Fat:	6.5g	**Fiber:**	10.7g	**Omega 6:**	0.6g
Protein:	10.4g	**Cholesterol:**	5mg	**Ratio:**	0.24:1

A low-calorie starter dish that can double as an entrée if there's any remaining leftover meat or beans, just throw them in the stew alongside the tomatoes! Contains a good macronutrient split across the board.

Benefits: Fiber, Prebiotics & Anti-Inflammatory
Value: $
Time: 1 Hour 10 mins
Serves: 4

Ingredients
Small Bunch Basil (5g)
1 Onion (110g)
2 Garlic Cloves
3 Zucchinis (588g)
4 Large Sweet Potatoes (650g)
2 X 14oz (400g) Cans Chopped Tomatoes
1 Tbsp Olive Oil
5 Tbsp (25g) Parmesan

Method

1. Quarter the zucchinis lengthways and then cut into chunks. Chop the onion, crush the garlic and cut the sweet potatoes into chunks. Tear the basil and finely grate the parmesan.

2. Heat the oil in a large frying pan over a medium heat. Add the onion and cook for about 10 mins until softened and starting to go golden brown. Add the garlic and cook for 5 mins more.

3. Add the zucchinis and cook for about 5 mins until starting to soften. Tip in the tomatoes and give everything a good stir. Simmer for 20 mins, then add the sweet potatoes and simmer for an additional 15-20 mins or until tomatoes are reduced and the zucchinis and potatoes are soft, then stir in the basil and Parmesan. Serve.

Mexican Penne with Avocado

Macronutrients & Omegas per Serving

Kcal:	682	**Carbs:**	101.2g	**Omega 3:**	0.2g
Fat:	21.2g	**Fiber:**	30.6g	**Omega 6:**	2.4g
Protein:	24.9g	**Cholesterol:**	3mg	**Ratio:**	0.07:1

A spicy pasta dish that can be tailored to your taste buds. Turn down the heat by switching the hot chili powder to medium, excluding the jalapeno and having additional tablespoons of yogurt. A large portion… or lunch leftovers!

Benefits: Fiber, Prebiotics and Probiotics
Value: $
Time: 30 mins
Serves: 2

Ingredients
1/2 Jalapeno Pepper
1/2 Lime
Handful Cilantro
1 Large Onion (140g)
1 Orange Bell Pepper (120g)
1 Avocado (200g)
2 Garlic Cloves
1 1/2 Cups (150g) Whole Wheat Penne
14oz (400g) Can Chopped Tomatoes
14oz (400g) Can Butter Beans
½ Tsp Cumin Seeds
1 Tsp Olive Oil
1 Tsp Ground Cilantro
1 Tsp Vegetable Bouillon Powder
2 Tsp Hot Chili Powder
2 Tbsp Greek Yogurt

Method

1. Finely chop 1 tbsp onion and then slice the rest. Deseed and cut the orange bell pepper into chunks. Slice the jalapeno (if using), grate the garlic, zest and juice 1/2 lime, stone, peel and chop the avocado and chop the cilantro.

2. Heat the oil in a medium pan. Add the sliced onion and pepper and fry, stirring frequently for 10 mins until golden. Stir in the garlic and spices, then tip in the tomatoes, half a can of water, the corn and bouillon. Cover and simmer for 15 mins.

3. Cook the pasta as per its instructions until al dente.

4. Meanwhile, toss the avocado with the lime juice and zest, and the finely chopped onion.

5. Drain the penne and toss into the sauce with the cilantro. Spoon the pasta into bowls, top with the avocado and jalapeno slices, scatter over the cilantro leaves and dollop of Greek yogurt.

Spicy Roast Veg & Lentils

Macronutrients & Omegas per Serving

Kcal:	675	**Carbs:**	114.1g	**Omega 3:**	0.3g
Fat:	13.1g	**Fiber:**	21.3g	**Omega 6:**	1.6g
Protein:	33.3g	**Cholesterol:**	0mg	**Ratio:**	0.17:1

Roasted vegetable dishes require lots of prep work, and then the hard work pays off when you throw it in the oven and relax. All of the veg and beans culminate into a very fibrous meal.

Benefits: Fiber and Prebiotics
Value: $
Time: 1 hour
Serves: 4

Ingredients
1 Red Onion (150g)
1 Small-Medium Butternut Squash (1lb/950g)
Large Handful Cilantro
2 Garlic Cloves
3 Bell Peppers (360g)
21oz (600g) Can Puy Lentils
5floz (150ml) Hot Vegetable Stock
3 Tbsp Olive Oil
3 Tbsp Curry Paste

Method
1. Using a sharp knife, peel the butternut squash. Cut it in half lengthways, scoop out the seeds, then cut into small-medium cubes. Halve and thickly slice the onion, deseed and cut the bell peppers into 0.5-inch (1cm) wide strips. Drain and rinse the lentils. Chop the cilantro and finely chop the garlic.

2. Heat oven to 400°F (200°C)/350°F (180°C) fan/gas 6. Put the squash cubes in a large roasting tin with the onion, and garlic. Mix the oil with the curry paste and drizzle over the vegetables. Toss well to coat in the curry mix and season.

3. Roast for 20 mins then add the peppers and roast for an additional 10 mins until the vegetables are beginning to soften.

4. Make the vegetable stock as per instructions or heat pre-made stock. Add the lentils and stock to the roasting tin and mix. Return to the oven for a further 5-10 mins until the vegetables are tender. Stir in the cilantro and serve immediately.

Prawn Jalfrezi

Macronutrients & Omegas per Serving

Kcal:	404	**Carbs:**	66.6g	**Omega 3:**	0.1g
Fat:	8.2g	**Fiber:**	9.7g	**Omega 6:**	1g
Protein:	21.3g	**Cholesterol:**	77mg	**Ratio:**	0.14:1

Nothing beats giant juicy prawns in a Jalfrezi. This humble Indian dish is greater than the sum of its parts, showcasing how the right mixture of spices create an aromatic sauce. If the sauce is too thick for your liking, add a few tablespoons of water.

Benefits: Fiber, Prebiotics and Probiotics
Value: $$$
Time: 35 mins
Serves: 2
Ingredients
1/2 Lemon
Small Bunch Cilantro
Thumb-Sized Piece Ginger (16g)
1 Large Green Bell Pepper (150g)
2 Onions (220g)
2 Garlic Cloves
8 Tiger Prawns (140g)
1 1/2 Cups Brown Rice (150g)
14oz (400g) Can Chopped Tomato
¼ Tsp Chili Flakes
½ Tsp Ground Turmeric
½ Tsp Ground Cumin
1 Tsp Ground Cilantro
2 Tsp Olive Oil
1 Tbsp Curry Paste
1 Tbsp Clear Honey
2 Tbsp Greek Yogurt

Method

1. Chop the onions and garlic then finely chop the ginger. Halve, deseed and chop the green bell pepper. Separate the stalks from the leaves of the cilantro and chop both. Squeeze the lemon juice into a bowl. Peel and clean the prawns. Cook the brown rice as per its instructions.

2. Heat the oil in a non-stick pan and fry the onions, ginger and garlic for 6 mins, stirring frequently, until softened and starting to color. If you've bought the prawns pre-cooked, skip this step and continue cooking the onions for 2 more mins, otherwise add the uncooked prawns, cook for an additional 2 mins then remove the prawns and set aside.

3. Add the spices and chili flakes, stir briefly, then pour in the tomatoes with the honey. Stir in the pepper, cilantro stalks and prawns. Cover the pan and leave to simmer for 5 mins, then add the prawns and simmer for an additional 5 mins. The mixture will be very thick and splutter a little, so stir frequently. The shrimps are cooked when they've shrunk in size and are no long shrinking, exterior is pink and flesh slightly white in color. If the flesh is bright white, the shrimps may be overcooked.

4. Scatter over the cilantro leaves. Serve the rice and prawn jalfrezi with Greek yogurt if you'd like.

Miso Brown Rice & Chicken Salad

Macronutrients & Omegas per Serving

Kcal:	380	**Carbs:**	42.8g	**Omega 3:**	0.1g
Fat:	7.6g	**Fiber:**	5.1g	**Omega 6:**	1.5g
Protein:	38g	**Cholesterol:**	87mg	**Ratio:**	0.06:1

Capitalizing on miso's probiotic profile, this quick rice dish provides an influx of good bacteria directly to the gut.

Benefits: Probiotics
Value: $$
Time: 45 mins
Serves: 2

Ingredients
2 Skinless Chicken Breasts (300g)
4 Scallions (60g)
1 1/2 Cups (150g) Brown Basmati Rice
5oz (140g) Sprouting Broccoli
2 Tsp Grated Ginger
4 Tsp Miso Paste
1 Tbsp Toasted Sesame Seeds
2 Tbsp Rice Vinegar
2 Tbsp Mirin

Method
1. Cook the rice as per its instructions then drain and keep warm. Cut the onions into diagonal slices.

2. Place the chicken breasts into a pan of boiling water so they are completely covered. Boil for 1 min, then turn off the heat, place a lid on and let it sit for 15 mins. When cooked through, cut into slices.

3. Boil the broccoli until tender. Drain, rinse under cold water and drain again.

4. For the dressing, mix the miso, rice vinegar, mirin and ginger together.

5. Divide the rice between two plates and scatter over the scallions and sesame seeds. Place the broccoli and chicken slices on top. To finish, drizzle over the dressing.

Barbequed Sweet Potatoes Filled with a Chickpea Spinach Salad

Macronutrients & Omegas per Serving

Kcal:	437	**Carbs:**	43.9g	**Omega 3:**	0.7g
Fat:	24.9g	**Fiber:**	11g	**Omega 6:**	5.5g
Protein:	11.1g	**Cholesterol:**	2mg	**Ratio:**	0.13:1

Time for a summer sweet potato treat! This dish has multiple levels of flavor; crispy potato skin, sweet potato, sour Greek yogurt tahini and juicy pomegranate seeds.

Benefits: Fiber and Probiotics
Value: $
Time: 1 hour 20
Serves: 4

Ingredients
Small Bunch Dill (5g)
1 Large Garlic Clove
1 Echalion Shallot (50g)
1 Lemon
4 Medium Sweet Potatoes (520g)
1/4 Cup (25g) Toasted Walnuts
2/3 Cup (110g) Pomegranate Seeds
2 1/2 Cups (75g) Baby Leaf Spinach
14oz (400g) Can Chickpeas
2 Tbsp Tahini
3 1/2 Tbsp Greek Yogurt
4 Tbsp Olive Oil

Method
1. Crush the garlic and finely chop the shallot and dill. Zest and Juice the lemon then drain the chickpeas.
2. Wrap each potato in foil and put directly on the hot coals of a barbecue for 35-45 mins, depending on the size of the potatoes. Insert

a skewer into each one to check that they're cooked. Alternatively, heat oven to 400°F (200°C)/350°F (180°C) fan/gas 6 and put the foil-wrapped potatoes on a large baking sheet. Bake in the oven for 45 mins-1 hour or until the center is soft. Once cooked, put under a hot grill for 3 mins until the skin is blackened and crispy.

3. After 20 mins of barbecuing the potatoes (or 35 mins of baking them), heat 1 tbsp olive oil in a large frying pan over a medium heat. Add the garlic and shallot and fry for 2-3 mins until softened, then stir the chickpeas into the mixture. Gently warm for 1 min, add the spinach and leave to wilt. Add the dill.

4. Whisk together the lemon juice, zest and 3 tbsp olive oil in a small bowl. Season to taste and stir into the chickpea mixture. Gently mash with a potato masher until the chickpeas are slightly crushed. Mix together the yogurt and tahini in another small bowl, and season to taste with salt.

5. Split the potatoes open lengthways. Fill with the bean mixture, drizzle over the tahini yogurt and top with the hazelnuts and pomegranate seeds.

Butternut Squash Casserole

Macronutrients & Omegas per Serving

Kcal:	334	**Carbs:**	60.1g	**Omega 3:**	0.1g
Fat:	8.8g	**Fiber:**	10.6g	**Omega 6:**	1g
Protein:	9.1g	**Cholesterol:**	2mg	**Ratio:**	0.1:1

An easy casserole that requires a lot of prep and then throwing in the oven, perfect for scaling to larger batches. Feel free to add additional chili powder to increase the heat, which will be offset by the yogurt.

Benefits: Fiber and Prebiotics
Value: $$
Time: 1 Hour
Serves: 4

Ingredients
1 Onion (110g)
1 Red Bell Pepper (120g)
1 Butternut Squash (550g)
2 Garlic Cloves
2 Sweet Potatoes (260g)
1/2 Cup (90g) Bulgur Wheat
14oz (400g) Can Chopped Tomato
17floz (500ml) Vegetable Stock
1 Tsp Cumin Seeds
2 Tbsp Olive Oil
2 Tbsp Paprika
4 Tbsp Greek Yogurt

Method

1. Slice the onion, crush the garlic, deseed and chop the bell pepper, peel the squash and then chop both the squash and sweet potatoes into small cubes.

2. In a large pan, heat the olive oil, then cook the onion and garlic for 5-7 mins until the onion is softened. Add the cumin seeds and paprika, then cook for a further 2 mins. Stir in the sweet potato, red bell pepper and butternut squash and toss with the onion and spices for 2 mins.

3. Pour in the tomatoes, vegetable stock, season, then simmer gently for 15 mins. Stir in the bulgur wheat, cover with a lid, then simmer for 15 mins more until the sweet potato and squash are tender, the bulgur wheat is cooked, and the liquid has been absorbed.

4. Serve in bowls topped with a spoonful of Greek yogurt.

Pumpkin and Chickpea Curry

Macronutrients & Omegas per Serving

Kcal: 554	**Carbs:** 57.6g	**Omega 3:** 0g
Fat: 31.9g	**Fiber:** 8.9g	**Omega 6:** 1.2g
Protein: 14.6g	**Cholesterol:** 1mg	**Ratio:** 0.03:1

Complemented by the coconut milk and assortment of spices, the Thai curry paste adds a heap load of flavor. If you don't have naan bread, substitute it with 3/4 cup of brown rice per person.

Benefits: Fiber and Prebiotics
Value: $
Time: 40 mins
Serves: 4

Ingredients
Large Handful Mint Leaves
1 Piece Pumpkin or Small Squash (35oz/1kg)
2 Whole Wheat Naan Bread (212g)
2 Limes
2 Onions (220g)
2 Large Stalks Lemongrass
6 Cardamom Pods
14oz (400g) Can Chickpeas
13.5floz (400ml) Can Coconut Milk
1/2 Tsp Chili Flakes
1 Tbsp Olive Oil
1 Tbsp Mustard Seed
3 Tbsp Yellow Thai Curry Paste

Method
1. Finely chop the onions and bash the lemongrass with the back of a knife. Drain and rinse the chickpeas. Dice the pumpkin or squash into small cubes.

2. Heat the oil in a sauté pan, then gently fry the curry paste with the onions, lemongrass, cardamom, chili flakes and mustard seed for 2-3 mins until fragrant. Stir the pumpkin or squash into the pan and coat in the paste, then pour in the stock and coconut milk. Bring everything to a simmer, add the chickpeas, then cook for about 10 mins until the pumpkin is tender, if using butternut squash this could take 15 mins depending on how small the cubes are.

3. Squeeze the juice of one lime into the curry, then cut the other lime into wedges to serve alongside. Just before serving, remove the lemongrass and tear over mint leaves, then bring to the table with the lime wedges and warm naan breads.

Teriyaki Salmon with Pak Choi

Macronutrients & Omegas per Serving

Kcal:	580	**Carbs:**	44.9g	**Omega 3:**	3.5g
Fat:	30.4g	**Fiber:**	2.7g	**Omega 6:**	2.6g
Protein:	32.6g	**Cholesterol:**	72mg	**Ratio:**	1.35:1

A succulent salmon fillet bathed in a teriyaki style sauce with one major change, no sesame oil, as it contains an extremely poor Omega 3 to Omega 6 ratio. This recipe goes to show that you can make simple substitutions that have little impact on flavor but big impact on health.

Benefits: Fiber, Prebiotics and Anti-inflammatory
Value: $$$
Time: 30 mins
Serves: 2

Ingredients
2 Skinless Salmon Fillets (260g)
3 Garlic Cloves
1 1/2 Cups (150g) Brown Rice
9oz (250g) Bok Choy
2 Tsp Grated Ginger
5 Tsp Olive Oil
1 Tbsp Sweet Chili Sauce
1 Tbsp Honey
1 Tbsp Mirin
2 Tbsp Soy Sauce

Method
1. Grate the ginger and garlic.

2. Heat the oven to 400°F (200°C)/350°F (180°C) fan/gas 6 and put 2 skinless salmon fillets in a shallow baking dish. Cook the brown rice as per its instructions.

3. Mix 1 tbsp sweet chili sauce, 1 tbsp honey, 1 tsp olive oil, 1 tbsp mirin or dry sherry, 2 tbsp soy sauce and 2 tsp finely grated ginger in a small bowl and pour over the salmon so the fillets are completely covered. Bake for 15-20 mins, to test if done, put a toothpick through the thickest part, if you feel resistance then it's still raw, if you feel no resistance then it's done.

3. Cut a slice across the base of 2 large bok choy so the leaves separate. Heat 4 tsp olive oil in a wok, add 3 grated garlic cloves and stir-fry briefly to soften, then add the bok choy and fry for 1-2 mins.

4. Serve the bok choy in shallow bowls, top with the salmon and spoon over the juices. Serve with brown rice.

Ground Beef & Sweet Potato Stew

Macronutrients & Omegas per Serving

Kcal:	532	**Carbs:**	36.7g	**Omega 3:**	0g
Fat:	34.3g	**Fiber:**	6.6g	**Omega 6:**	0.5g
Protein:	21.4g	**Cholesterol:**	86mg	**Ratio:**	0.07:1

A hearty winter stew which is perfect for scaling up and freezing. Sweet potato brings the fiber and the Worcestershire sauce and bouillon brings the tangy flavor.

Benefits: Fiber and Prebiotics
Value: $$
Time: 1 hour 20
Serves: 4

Ingredients
Few Thyme Sprigs
Handful Parsley
1 Large Onion (140g)
1 Large Carrot (75g)
1 Celery Stick (40g)
1 Beef Bouillon Cube
1 Bay Leaf
14oz (400g) Can Chopped Tomato
1lb (450g) Ground Beef
1lb (450g) Sweet Potatoes
1 Tbsp Olive Oil
1 Tbsp Tomato Purée
1 Tbsp Worcestershire Sauce

Method
1. Chop the onion, carrot and parsley, slice the celery stick. Cut the sweet potato into large chunks.

2. Heat the oil in a large pan, add the onion, carrot and celery, and cook on low heat for 10 mins, stirring frequently until soft. Add the beef and cook until it is browned all over.

3. Add the tomato purée and cook for a few mins, then add the Worcestershire sauce, tomatoes, sweet potatoes, herbs, can full of water and bouillon cube. Bring to the boil.

4. Simmer on a low heat for 40-45 mins until the sweet potatoes are tender, stirring a few times throughout cooking to make sure they are cooking evenly.

5. Once cooked, remove the bay leaf, stir through the chopped parsley and serve with cabbage.

Conclusion

If you or someone close to you is suffering from diverticulosis or diverticulitis attacks it can be emotionally and physically damaging. However, you are not alone. Although we do not currently know the exact reason behind why diverticulosis occurs, lack of fiber and consistent straining or constipation seem to be a reoccurring trigger. It is interesting that western people are much more susceptible to these conditions. This is often attributed to genes or differences in diet.

The amount of people that will develop diverticulosis in their lifetimes is astonishing. Although this disease is currently incurable, there are many alternative methods that can reduce the suffering and prevent diverticulosis from turning into diverticulitis. Increasing fiber intake, consuming foods with anti-inflammatory properties such as fish, restoring intestinal flora with probiotics and reducing stress by taking up stress management activities such as meditation or yoga can ease the symptoms of diverticular disease and prevent diverticulitis.

As digestive disorders are becoming more frequent, so is the attention the medical community gives towards this field. So, I urge you to take your health seriously, adopt lifestyle changes and focus on your eating habits so as to prevent a diverticulitis attack. Most people with diverticulosis will never experience any serious symptoms that wouldn't otherwise be mistaken as indigestion. Hopefully we can keep it that way. By taking small but consistent dietary changes you may be able to prevent diverticulitis. As more time goes on, we are more likely to understand the causes and treatments but, in the meantime, I wish you good health.

Printed in Great Britain
by Amazon